New Trends of
Psychiatry in
the Community

New Trends of Psychiatry in the Community

Edited by
George Serban, M.D.

Foreword by
Boris Astrachan, M.D.

Ballinger Publishing Company • Cambridge, Massachusetts
A Subsidiary of J.B. Lippincott Company

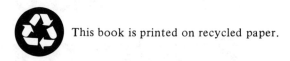 This book is printed on recycled paper.

Proceedings of the Fourth International Symposium of the Kittay Scientific Foundation, entitled "A Critical Appraisal of Community Psychiatry" held March 28–29, 1976, New York, N.Y.

Symposium sponsored by Kittay Scientific Foundation
S. Kittay, President
A. Zimmerman, Director of Communication

International Standard Book Number: 0–88410–516–4

Library of Congress Catalog Card Number: 77–6322

Printed in the United States of America

Library of Congress Cataloging in Publication Data

Main entry under title:

New trends of psychiatry in the community.

   1. Social psychiatry—Congresses. 2. Community mental health services—Congresses. 3. Epidemiology—Congresses. 4. Psychology, Pathological—Etiology—Congresses. I. Serban, George, 1926–
II. Kittay Scientific Foundation.
RC455.N44   362.2   77–6322
ISBN 0–88410–516–4

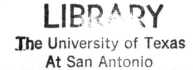

Contents

List of Figures

List of Tables

List of Authors

George Serban, M.D.
Associate Clinical Professor
   of Psychiatry
New York University
   Medical Center

Louis Jolyon West, M.D.
Professor and Chairman
Department of Psychiatry,
U.C.L.A.

Melvin Sabshin, M.D.
Medical Director
American Psychiatric Association

Prof. Dr. Pierre Pichot
Professor and Chairman
Department of Psychiatry
University of Paris
Paris, France

Frank Ochberg, M.D.
Director
Division of Mental Health Services
   Programs
National Institute of Mental Health

Lucy Ozarin, M.D.
Assistant Director for Program
   Development
Division of Mental Health Service
   Programs
National Institute of Mental Health

Stanley Yolles, M.D.
Professor and Chairman
Department of Psychiatry
State University of New York
   at Stony Brook

Alexander Leighton, M.D.
National Health Scientist (Canada)
Professor of Psychiatry and
   Preventive Medicine
Dalhousie University
Professor Emeritus, Harvard University

Bruce Dohrenwend, Ph.D.
Professor of Social Science
Department of Psychiatry
Social Psychiatry Research Unit
Columbia University

Thomas Langner, Ph.D.
Professor of Clinical Psychiatry
Division of Epidemiology
Columbia University

Joanne C. Gersten, Ph.D.
Associate Professor of Public Health
Division of Epidemiology
Columbia University

Jeanne G. Eisenberg, M.A.
Senior Staff Associate
Division of Epidemiology
Columbia University

Leo Srole, Ph.D.
Chief of Psychiatric Research,
    Social Sciences
New York State Psychiatric Institute
Extraordinary Professor of Faculty
    of Psychiatry and Education
Catholic University of Leuven
    (Louvaine) Belgium
Professor of Social Sciences
Department of Psychiatry
College of Physicians and Surgeons
Columbia University

Elmer L. Struening, Ph.D.
Director
Epidemiology of Mental Disorders Unit
New York State Department
    of Mental Hygiene

Martin Katz, M.D., Ph.D.
Chief, Clinical Research Branch
American College of Neuropsychology
National Institute of Mental Health

Loren R. Mosher, M.D.
Chief
Center for the Study of Schizophrenia
National Institute of Mental Health

Gary Tischler, M.D.
Professor of Clinical Psychiatry
Department of Psychiatry
Yale University School of Medicine

Robert B. Ellsworth, Ph.D.
Research Psychologist,
    Veterans Administration Hospital,
Salem, Virginia

Thomas Kiresuk, Ph.D.
Chief Clinical Psychologist
Hennepin County Medical Center

Sander Lund, M.A.
Coordinator
Program Evaluation Project
University of Minnesota Hospital

Ira Glick, M.D.
Associate Professor
Langley Porter Institute
University of California

Gerald Klerman, M.D.
Professor of Psychiatry
Massachusetts General Hospital
Harvard Medical School

William T. Carpenter, Jr., M.D.,
Director, Schizophrenia Research
Department of Psychiatry
Albert Einstein College of Medicine

Ernest Gruenberg, M.D.
Professor and Chairman
Department of Mental Hygiene
Johns Hopkins University
School of Hygiene & Public Health

Lawrence C. Kolb, M.D.
Chairman of the International
    Advisory Board
Commissioner, New York State
    Department of Mental Hygiene
Professor of Psychiatry,
    Columbia University

List of Participants

Boris Astrachan, M.D.
Director
Community Mental Health Center
Professor of Clinical Psychiatry
Yale University School of Medicine

Viola W. Barnard, M.D.
Former Director
Division of Community and Social
  Psychiatry
Former Clinical Professor of Psychiatry
College of Physicians and Surgeons
Columbia University

Francis J. Braceland, M.D.
Editor in Chief
The American Journal of Psychiatry
Senior Consultant
The Institute of Living

Archangelo Calobrisi, M.D.
Director of Psychiatry
Cabrini Health Care Center

Robert Cancro, M.D.
Professor of Psychiatry
University of Connecticut Health
  Center
Department of Psychiatry

Leonard Cook, Ph.D.
Director, Department of Pharmacology
Hoffman-LaRoche, Inc.

Prof. Dr. Börje Cronholm
Director
Department of Psychiatry
Karolinska Institute
Stockholm, Sweden

Barbara Dohrenwend, Ph.D.
Professor of Psychology
Department of Psychology
City College of the City University
  of New York

Alfred Freedman, M.D.
Professor & Chairman, Department
  of Psychiatry
New York Medical College

Fritz A. Freyhan, M.D.
Editor-in-Chief
Comprehensive Psychiatry
Editor-in-Chief
International Pharmacopsychiatry

J.L. Hakes, M.D.
Director of Clinical Research
Pfizer, International

Marvin Herz, M.D.
Director of Community Services
New York State Psychiatric Institute
Associate Professor
Clinical Psychiatry
College of Physicians and Surgeons
Columbia University

Donald F. Klein, M.D.
Director of Research and Evaluation
Hillside Hospital
Professor of Psychiatry
New York State University College
  of Medicine at Stony Brook

Heinz Lehmann, M.D.
Director of Medical Education
  and Research
Douglas Hospital
Montreal, Canada
Professor of Psychiatry
McGill University

Gilbert Levin, M.D.
Associate Professor of Psychiatry
  & Community Health
Department of Psychiatry
Albert Einstein College of Medicine
  of Yeshiva University

Dr. Theodore Lidz, M.D.
Professor of Psychiatry
Yale University
School of Medicine

Prof. Dr. Juan Lopez-Ibor
Chairman
Department of Psychiatry
University of Madrid
Madrid, Spain

Sidney Malitz, M.D.
Professor and Acting Chairman
Department of Psychiatry
Columbia University
Acting Director, New York State
  Psychiatric Institute

Robert Michels, M.D.
Professor of Psychiatry
Cornell University Medical Center
Psychiatrist-in-Chief
The New York Hospital

Prof. Dr. Pierre Pichot
Professor and Chairman
Department of Psychiatry
University of Paris
Paris, France

Jan Schrievers, M.D.
Co-Director
Geel Project, University of Leuven
Geel, Belgium

Robert A. Senescu, M.D.
Director
Department of Psychiatry
Beth Israel Medical Center

Foreword

Boris M. Astrachan, M.D.

The conference reported upon in this volume reflects an attempt to clarify the definition of community psychiatry, to identify its scientific roots, and to examine its clinical responsibilities. In the past, discussion of community psychiatry has been frustrated by the multiple definitions of the term, and dispute about tasks.

For many, the term connotes a social movement and the activities attendant upon such a phenomenon. Community psychiatry is equated with the Community Mental Health Movement of the 1960s. It is associated with the development of active consumerism, shifting bases of political power, some devaluation of intensive psychological work with patients, loss of confidence in professionals, an emphasis on nonspecific modes of prevention and social activism, and the development of new roles for allied health professionals as well as role blurring. This use of the term ignores history, links clinical practice to a social movement, and, to some extent, separates practice from its underlying scientific bases. Depending upon one's orientation, community psychiatry is, in this definition, either a force for needed change in the profession or a challenge to concepts of good patient care.

A second definition identifies community psychiatry as synonymous with a service delivery strategy. Under federal impetus, the settings of practice are extended into new institutional forms that deliver mandated services to defined population groups. Emphases are placed upon enhancing the availability and accessibility of service and upon the acceptance of responsibility for the mental health needs of the total population resident within a specified area. Initially, community mental health centers were required to provide inpatient, outpatient, partial hospitalization, and emergency services and consultation and education to community groups. The emphasis was upon clinical treatment structures and the provision of a range of services to meet patient needs.

In addition to the original list of mandated services, federal law now has added transitional treatment facilities (halfway houses), as well as categorical services for particular population groups: children, the aged, those discharged from inpatient settings, and the drug and alcohol addicted. The identification of community psychiatry with an organizational strategy, without clear definition of clinical tasks, at best promotes useful dialogue in regard to the integration of multiple approaches to care, and at worst stimulates conflict among medical and nonmedical approaches to care.

A.K. Rice [1, 2] has insisted that organizational structures ought to reflect organizational task. In mental health institutions clarity about task has not preceded definition of structures. My colleagues and I have identified four major task areas for psychiatry as a profession [3]. These include medical tasks, rehabilitative tasks, social control of deviancy tasks, and humanistic tasks. These task areas are interrelated but can be historically differentiated, reflect different value systems, require differing educational experiences for preparation of practitioners, and logically require differing interprofessional role relationships and organizational structures. Currently, there is only limited congruence between organizational structures and professional tasks. Thus we see this second definition as leading to premature definition of structure and inflexibility of practice.

The Kittay Scientific Foundation's Symposium on "A Critical Appraisal of Community Psychiatry" implicitly accepted a third definition of the term. Community psychiatry is identified as the best possible clinical care delivered to individuals and to population groups in community settings. Services are delivered in communities and their institutions rather than within the setting of total institutions (state hospitals, asylums, etc.). The emphasis is upon the major psychiatric disorders, particularly the schizophrenias and the affective disorders. Concern is focused upon the importance of identifying appropriate medical and rehabilitative resources in order to reduce patient symptoms, preserve functioning, and, where possible, enhance adaptation. This approach permits a more dispassionate and carefully focused inquiry into the body of knowledge and theory upon which psychiatric practice in the community might be based.

In this conference, the bases for practice are identified as residing in epidemiology and in clinical research.

The historical context and various definitions of community psychiatry are presented in the volume. Drawing upon his leadership experiences at NIMH, Yolles describes the development of mental health services through community mental health centers. Ochberg and Ozarin present a historical account of the community mental health movement and its influence upon the development of centers. These two papers describe community psychiatry within the contexts of social movement, and structural strategy. Srole describes the historical continuity of Gheel, a village in Belgium which has served as a therapeutic setting for the severely ill for over five centuries. He demonstrates that community "mental health" programming historically has been tied to clinical practice.

The importance of epidemiological research to clinical practice is thoroughly documented in the paper by Bruce and Barbara Dohrenwend. They summarize research strategies for evaluating the place of stress in the production of mental disorder. Their work extends and enlarges the researches of Leighton and others in providing data for the identification of rational bases for prevention. Langner's paper identifies a similar research strategy for examining the correlates of psychological distress in children. His ten-year study emphasizes the importance of stress in the production of psychological disorder in children.

Tischler's paper bridges epidemiological strategies and the area of clinical practice. He demonstrates the way in which epidemiology can be applied to understanding important issues in the delivery of services. Comparing data from service delivery systems to population sample data is an important contribution to methodology and to the design of treatment settings. The papers by Mosher and Ellsworth both identify and make use of clinical evaluation strategies to examine the processes and outcomes of clinical care.

In the final section, both Serban and Klerman identify the problems of those with schizophrenic illnesses. Klerman's review of clinical research studies is valuable both to clinicians and to those involved in the development of public policy. Serban's research emphasizes that many schizophrenic patients have a chronic course, and that medical care must be combined with rehabilitative and social services to meet patient needs. Both authors emphasize the importance of research to clinical practice and the development of policy.

At the symposium, these papers were discussed energetically by investigators and clinicians. A major intent was to develop recommendations for continued work, and to identify clinical and research priorities. The recommendations of the symposium centered on improving psychiatric treatment. The presenters and discussants accepted no current structures or treatment strategies as immutable. They insisted that prevention and improved treatment will depend upon clarity of task definition, greater understanding of disorders and disease, and increasingly sophisticated intervention strategies.

President Kennedy's message to Congress in 1963 stimulated public interest in mental illness and mental health and provided for treatment settings which have increased the accessibility and availability of service. Yet, even today, the mentally ill remain feared and isolated. Research is relatively poorly supported and resources for professional manpower development have been cut. A clear conclusion of the seminar is that the health of community psychiatry depends upon the excellence of psychiatric practice. Its continuing growth requires enhanced understanding of the major psychiatric disorders, clarity in regard to the tasks of the profession, and appropriate support.

New Trends of
Psychiatry in
the Community

Introduction

It is almost impossible for a week to go by without reading about another violent drama in which a discharged patient from a mental hospital is involved. On the other hand, the present government hearing regarding the poor treatment in foster homes for the mentally ill discharged into the community, brings into the open the reality concerning conditions offered to them by the community itself.

It appears that the new form of treatment—particularly, tranquilizers for the mentally disturbed—led to a change of our policy towards the institutionalization of these patients. Free from acute mental symptoms, they are let loose in the community. What has become evident is the fact that the majority do not integrate into their community or that the community is unable to absorb and accept them. There seems to be a missing link in the continuity of care of the mental patient at the time of his discharge from the hospital to his functional integration into the community, which is the responsibility of the local mental health service. This improper condition appears to affect not only the well being of the patient, but that of the community itself. This is the problem which I hope this distinguished gathering of scientists will be able to answer in these two days involved in working together and exchanging ideas.

I am told that between 3.5 to 10.0 percent of our population present one form or another of mental disorder; if these individuals live freely in our community with various degrees of mental symptoms are they helped to get better, to live more or less a normal life; if they are not, is the community protected from any of their harmful acts? From what I understand neither issue is clarified. For me as a businessman, I cannot help but think that if the maintenance of four million mentally ill patients costs the government more than five billion dollars a year, then what should be the results which justify this spending? From what you know at this time of mental illness, can our present mental health policies be documented scientifically and, if not, what can be done to improve them beyond academic rhetoric?

The concern of the public regarding the adequacy of the services offered to the emotionally disturbed, as supported by the press, shows the magnitude of the task faced by all of you, and the sense of urgency with which the problem should be treated.

As President of the Kittay Scientific Foundation, I wish you success in your endeavor to find better solutions to this intolerable and disturbing human condition, which affects every human being in the community.

Sol Kittay

Objectives of the Symposium

George Serban

Community psychiatry, imported from Europe together with tranquilizers, has progressively grown into a big and lucrative business with humanitarian overtones. Caught in the social turmoil of the sixties, it became another symbol for the liberation of the oppressed minority of the mentally ill at this time. Supported by scanty social evidence produced by fragmented social research, community psychiatry became used by social activists, self-styled "guardians for the rights of the mentally ill," as springboards for personal political objectives.

The alleged correlation between mental illness and social class became the justification for attempts to replace the medical model with the social political one, which allegedly would have cured not only the social imperfection of society but also our mental illness. Even the Russians, who deny the existence of a social conflict in their society, would not have accepted this formulation to the extent to which they believe in a biological basis for mental disorders.

The enthusiasm of the sixties was expressed by massive, indiscriminate discharge of mental patients from the hospitals, when every psychiatrist believed himself to be a "new Pinel" making history. This situation was replaced by the sober realism of the seventies. After the "revolving door policy" instituted in the sixties, the profession started to question the wisdom of unselective discharge of mental patients into the community, while the community, unable to absorb the chronic mentally ill, appeared to be somewhat reluctant to take care of them.

The catchword of the sixties, "liberation of mentally ill from protective detention," became replaced in the seventies by treatment in the least restrictive programs. Yet here is the problem. The programs are less restricted for whom? For the patient who doesn't want treatment, or for the community who cannot force the patient to receive it? While the social model of mental illness would like the community to accept the mentally ill regardless, since his illness is produced by the social system; this model has failed to find a solution to patients' integration into the community, or at least failed to take responsibility for his antisocial acts.

The responsibility for patients' social misbehavior remains with the psychiatrist and his institution. The controversy runs unabated, with psychiatrists defending each position according to their vested interest and knowledge. In this context, this outstanding group of scientists has a difficult task: to recommend solutions that will advance our possibilities of helping the mentally ill under the best available conditions, for the purpose of rehabilitation and reintegration into the community.

The objectives of this symposium are related to debating what are the valid factors helpful for the consolidation of community psychiatry, and what could be the necessary innovations and corrections for the improvement of its efficiency. The first question to be asked in this respect refers to its rationale. Based on the experience of the sixties, we know that approximately 15 percent of chronic patients are refractory regarding treatment, subsequently deteriorate and cannot be maintained in the community on a regular basis. We know as well that voluntary treatment in the community leads to multiple rehospitalizations due to patients' lack of interest and treatment. The New York State Task Force on Criteria for Admissions and Readmissions has recently presented some palliative solutions which, if they can be truly implemented, raise another set of problems about their ability to solve the issue.

The second set of questions are raised related to primary and secondary prevention of mental disorders. There is a general consensus that stressful familial or societal interaction leads to emotional disturbance in some individuals of particular genetic disposition. If this is so, how would these possible findings be included in the prevention and treatment of the mentally ill?

Another set of data has to deal with the evaluation of mental health service and its efficacy for the adjustment of the patient in the community. Are our measurements a good index of patients' adjustment, or are they based on all types of clinical inventories, unable to tap the real functioning of patients at the community level.

Finally, but not less important, regarding the appraisal of our realistic possibilities and our limitations in helping the emotionally disturbed, we must attempt to separate as much as possible those groups of mentally ill (particularly schizophrenics) who can be helped in the community from those who cannot. In this area, positive social and individual factors should be identified in terms of their contribution to the eventual adjustment of patients in the community.

This is not an easy task, particularly when our knowledge is fragmented, incomplete, and sometimes contradictory. Yet, by giving full weight to these facts, our claims should be more modest and documented. As long as our projections are hyperbolic, the public will continue to hold us responsible for cure or control of behavior disorders with regard to the mentally ill in the community—which in fact we can neither master, predict, nor understand, except through hindsight.

Setting the Problem

Louis Jolyon West

There are four million individuals in the United States who can be deemed mentally ill, and we ask ourselves how to justify spending $5 billion a year on their care. Thus we not only have indicated the fact that there is a large problem in the population, and a considerable expense, but have translated into individual daily costs to about $3.65 per patient per day. Then the question must be asked, what can be done for four million sick people by spending $3.65 a day per patient for their care?

Different solutions have been offered recently through redefinitions of the problem. One way of redefining the problem is by looking at a goodly number of these four million people and saying, well, they're not really mentally ill at all, and therefore we don't have to spend any money on them. Another way of looking at the problem is to say that the nature of mental illness is not that closely related to medical care, and therefore shouldn't be that closely related to medical costs. Those of us who have had anything to do with medical care for physical illness would agree that $3.65 a day wouldn't go very far.

Now, as we look at this issue in the context of the recent political situation, we see some strange conflicts between fiscal realities and medical ideals. An example can be seen in the State of California. During the tenure of a recent governor, a strange combination of factors resulted in some remarkable actions. A fiscally conservative executive seized eagerly upon proposals by the putative leadership of community mental health forces in the state, to the effect that patients would be better treated in their own communities than in psychiatric hospitals operated (at considerable cost) by the state. The consequence was a widespread shutting down of hospitals, thereby satisfying the parties on both sides. The enthusiasts of community mental health hailed the idea of more treatment and care of patients in the community, with diminution of the loss of individual freedom through hospitalization. The fiscally conservative leadership in the executive branch was delighted because the change was going to represent a substantial savings through the reduction of hospital costs.

I don't need to tell this group what the net result proved to be. We're all familiar with it. Patients were dumped back into communities which did not really possess the necessary resources to provide high quality local care. Local care, if it is to be comparable to the care delivered by even a moderately good mental hospital, is probably going to be more expensive, rather than less expensive, in terms of patient daily cost. This is simply because such care must be more individualized.

The community mental health movement in this country, historically speaking, was not a consequence or even an accompaniment of the psychopharmacological revolution. But the fact that these two major changes in the field of psychiatry took place during the same brief era (roughly 1950–1975) has obscured some of the scientific and social issues relating to both. There were lessons to be learned about the limitations of what we would now call community mental health, going back to Europe in the 1930s and even before. But if we look primarily at the postwar period in this country, prior to the development of the tranquilizing drugs and some of the other newer medications, there were two other important trends.

The first was a tremendous interest in psychiatry as a field. During and after World War II this led to a marked increase in the number of training opportunities and the interest in dynamic psychiatry within the medical profession itself. This phase was largely dominated by psychoanalytic thinking, but it had an effect far broader than that which could be measured by the production of more psychoanalysts.

The second came after the Korean conflict, and is probably best represented by the achievements of Col. Albert J. Glass of the United States Army, who was able to demonstrate in Korea some lessons of combat psychiatry from World War II and even World War I. He emphasized that patients were best cared for as close to the front (the site of the development of their symptoms) as possible. He showed that the sooner patients were returned to what was for them "normal" circumstances (even though those circumstances included the hazards of combat), the more advantageous it would be in terms of long term consequences for their mental health and subsequent treatment outcome.

Dr. Glass got the Gorgas Medal, and the Korean conflict was soon forgotten. But the lessons of Korea weren't so soon forgotten as was traditional after previous conflicts. And in those days, the early fifties, the roots of the present community mental health movement were firmly established.

Now it will be difficult but necessary for us to tease apart what the overlay of the psychopharmacological explosion did to the sociomedical process represented by President Kennedy's "bold new approach." His national campaign for community mental health began in the early 1960s, coming out of the plans and procedures that were already laid out (mainly at the National Institute of Mental Health) going back into the middle and late fifties. There would have been a "revolving door" phenomenon in the mental hospitals in any case as a consequence of the discovery of major tranquilizers, even if there had been no community mental health movement. This was simply because it became *possible* to get people out of the hospital and sent somewhere else. When they did get out, it was likely that many of them would encounter stress, or stop taking their medication, and have to come back.

We can't blame the "revolving door" upon the community mental health development. What we can do however is to ask ourselves three questions.

1. Given that in the 1950s and '60s there was a great national interest in the problems of the mentally ill—and also a great national belief in the power of psychiatry and the allied fields to do something about it—was a national policy to develop community mental health programs the best investment we could have made with available resources at that time? Several billions of dollars were spent during the golden years of the National Institute of Mental Health in its efforts to develop programs oriented largely to the idea of community mental health centers. These centers were to have substance of their own. They were in essence to be independent or semi-independent. The man who was responsible for administering the majority of NIMH funds during that period of time was Dr. Stanley Yolles.

But these questions were already being asked by Dr. Yolles and his advisers during those exciting years. A national commitment had been made long before Dr. Yolles took administrative charge of the National Institute of Mental Health. Now, in retrospect, would this enormous investment have been better if, for example, the funds had been employed in an effort to provide a sound psychiatric service in every community general hospital? What would have happened if the psychiatric developments of the 1960s had been more closely grafted onto the major developments in the field of health as a whole? I'm talking now about comprehensive community general hospitals, including psychiatry, instead of separate comprehensive community mental health programs.

Of course this must be seen in the context of the 1950s, when it was thought by many that the medical profession was never likely to accept such a close relationship to psychiatry and to the care of the mentally ill. Nevertheless we are entitled to ask ourselves now whether or not the funds that went into the community mental health movement might have done more good in the long run, if they had gone to develop psychiatric services in general hospitals instead.

2. The second question that we're entitled to ask ourselves is whether the investment that was made as part of the community mental health movement, to develop a great many paramedical or nonmedical helpers for the mentally ill, would have been better invested into medical education and a transformation of the medical profession itself. We know that enormous sums were spent during this period of time on a variety of activities that had to do essentially with upgrading patient care programs both in mental hospitals and in community programs. A relatively small amount actually went into medical education as such. And even in medical education proper, the least significant investment was made in undergraduate medical teaching.

Now, if we had made a substantially larger investment in the education of every physician, emphasizing mental health issues including the major mental illnesses, psychosomatic and psychophysiological problems, and psychosocial consequences or ramifications of mental illness, could we not have changed the whole shape of the medical profession by now? If so, every physician would be far more of a psychiatrist than he presently is, and all the power and all of the influence of the entire medical profession would today be more closely addressed to the mental health issues of the community as a whole than is presently the case.

3. Finally, I must pose the toughest question of the three. What should have been the appropriate relationship between investment in the application of existing knowledge during the 1950s and '60s, and investment in the development of new knowledge? Research was seen as important, but nevertheless it had to compete with community mental health programs and mental health service delivery pro-

grams for funding and for support. The idea of developing research people and research programs on a large scale nationally, and maintaining these people and programs through thick and thin, was recognized as important from the very beginning of our bold new national commitment to mental health in the postwar era.

Yet I think it is fair to say that of all aspects of our contemporary psychiatric milieu, the aspect least related to research—the one which seems to have developed the fewest tough-minded investigators and produced the least new knowledge—was the community mental health aspect of the total mental health commitment of the country.

These three questions are not easy to answer. But they have preoccupied many of us for the past 25 years. I hope that the deliberations here, especially as presented by people who are much closer to finding the answers to these questions than I have ever been, will be illuminating to us all.

Opening Remarks

Melvin Sabshin

It is certainly my privilege to join this symposium and to offer greetings from the APA (American Psychiatric Association). I do indeed believe that the International Symposia, sponsored and planned under the auspices of the Kittay Scientific Foundation, have become major events for psychiatry on a worldwide level, and I congratulate all of you who have provided the ideas and the resources for these meetings. This year's topic has specific significance and timeliness, and I am pleased that you have facilitated a reappraisal of community psychiatry. My comments on the subject are personal opinions and not necessarily a reflection of APA policies.

It is somewhat fashionable now in the United States to be critical of community and social psychiatry. At the international level there are significant transnational differences in the historical development and the current status of community psychiatry. I did have an opportunity at a recent World Psychiatric Association symposium on Primary Prevention to note these variations in attitudes and approaches. In any case, in the United States it is now more fashionable to be critical than in almost any other country. In part, the criticism is still based on ideological perspectives. Perhaps even more cogently, some of the criticism is based on concern over cost benefits; while some data is available it is so sparse that clear-cut conclusions are not easily forthcoming.

In my judgment, the most vocal criticism reflects new and emerging force fields in the United States. Community psychiatry was at the crest of the psychiatric wave of the 1960s. It indeed symbolized,

13

epitomized and in many ways was at the vanguard of the dominant psychiatric themes of the 1960s. To rectify disparity in psychiatric care by social class was the major motif and in some cases the leading slogan of that decade. Community psychiatry was perceived by many as the system to reduce the disparity. Similar to many other fields and developments in the United States during the decade of 1962–1972, community psychiatry became associated with pragmatism, eclecticism and a tendency for boundary expansionism.

There is a book that needs to be written on a comparative analysis of multiple social movements in health, education, welfare and even the governance of big cities in the United States. The author of that as-yet-unwritten monograph should compare some of the hopes and aspirations of the 1960s with the realities of the 1970s. As community psychiatry struggled for survival, it tended in many quarters to become increasingly antideterministic, anti-intellectual, and anti-scientific. To get on with the task was more important than appraising the work conducted heretofore.

Now the scene has changed dramatically; coping with new accountabilities is the psychiatric slogan of the 1970s in the United States, and indeed in several other countries also. Boundary building has replaced expansionism in psychiatry. There is even a tendency in some quarters to move 180 degrees opposite to the dominant themes of the 1960s. Social psychiatry has assumed a negative context for many psychiatric colleagues, and in part their pejorative attitude is a reaction to the excesses of the 1960s, including role diffusion as experienced by psychiatrists.

Critical appraisal of community psychiatry, the title of this symposium in the context of the new wave of the latter 1970s, led by ideologues who represent the new wave, has the danger of becoming a euphemism for a witch hunt rather than a scientifically responsible act. Hopefully this symposium has already and will continue to reflect neither the extreme passionate fervor of the 1960s nor the malignant counterreaction of the 1970s. Rather I would hope that there is a scientific spirit at this symposium that might take a careful look and thus help to create a new balanced approach; a new balance in which there is clear understanding of the hopes, expectations and aspirations of the previous decade.

In that context there should be an effort to assess not only the process and the outcome of community efforts, but of all other therapeutic intervention in this same spirit. These assessments need to be conducted with an eye to effectiveness, including cost effectiveness, an area where we have remained somewhat sluggish in the past. There is a need for clinical evaluations with emphasis on quality assurance and utilizing comparative analytic techniques across institutions, across geographic areas within the United States, and indeed ultimately on an international level. Such clinical studies need broad public and professional support.

We professionals must demonstrate an awareness of the need for responsible actions on our part by helping to develop a system that requires *appropriate* accountability. We need to provide responsible answers to the sympathetic critics who ask for our data or at least we must demonstrate a willingness to collect data. If the spirit of objective inquiry, coupled with an awareness of the needs for service, dominate this symposium, and the ideas and recommendations to implement new approaches flow in the same style, then I believe that the symposium can make a major contribution.

Chapter 1

Pierre Pichot (Moderator)

The Rationale of Community Mental Health

Frank M. Ochberg
Lucy D. Ozarin

The Kittay symposium comes at an opportune time, for we are about to launch a broadened and more extensive community mental health center program in the United States. This meeting, which is evaluating the theory and practice of community mental health, will provide guidelines to the effort.

The community mental health center is an organizational form through which community mental health principles are being put into practice in this country. The symposium asks, "What is the rationale?" Congress has provided its rationale in PL 94−63, Title III of which is the Community Mental Health Center Amendments of 1975. The law states (Sec. 302):

(1) community mental health care is the most effective and humane form of care for a majority of mentally ill individuals;

(2) the federally funded community mental health centers have had a major impact on the improvement of mental health care by—

(A) fostering coordination and cooperation between various agencies responsible for mental health care which, in turn, has resulted in a decrease in overlapping services and more efficient utilization of available resources.

(B) bringing comprehensive community mental health care to all in need within a specific geographic area regardless of ability to pay, and

(C) developing a system of care which insures continuity of care for all patients,

and thus are a national resource to which all Americans should enjoy access.

In 1973, the Government Accounting Office (GAO), after investigation of the federally funded community mental health program, reported to Congress, "The centers have increased the accessibility, quality and type of community services available and have enhanced the responsiveness of mental health services to individual needs. Some success has also been realized in mobilizing State and local resources to further program objectives" [1, p. 1]. The report helps identify several administrative and accounting deficiencies and the obvious need to further develop relationships with state hospitals.

The joint Congress and GAO report provides the political and legislative rationale for the national community mental health program. This symposium was prepared to appraise the movement critically from a scientific standpoint. This may not be a simple task because of the multiple and complex variables involved. Community mental health appears to be based on a dynamic interplay between social and cultural forces on the one hand and scientific knowledge on the other. Marmor applies general systems theory to community psychiatry, conceiving of mental health and illness as "resultants of a concentric network of interconnected determinants with the individual at the core of the network but in a constant state of dynamic interaction with elements related to family, peer groups, social class and larger community, as well as with ethnic, social, economic, and cultural subsystems" [2, p. 808]. Community psychiatry sees mental disorder as residing not just within the individual but also in disturbances within this dynamic network of interactive systems.

Thomas and Garrison develop the general systems view of community mental health further. They note that the community mental health movement

> emerged in the 1960s out of a confluence of historical trends and events. . . . The CMHC is clearly a structure in transition between a mental hospital and something else, the outlines of which are only emerging. . . . The theory and practice of psychiatry in the public sector are also clearly in transition from the earlier narrow medical and custodial models of treatment of the mentally ill in isolated "total institutions" to something else, the outlines of which are even less clear [3, p. 265].

They believe that a reconceptualization of community mental health in a general systems model is required and that systems science avoids the pitfalls of polarities. They foresee the blending of the clinical and social aspects of health and illness into one system based on a comprehensive set of theories to guide community mental health action.

THE HISTORICAL CONTEXT

Community mental health evolved from deep historic roots. Primitive attitudes toward the mentally ill caused them to be burned as witches, banished as paupers, or venerated as oracles. Albert Deutsch recounted such history in this country up to the end of World War II [4]. He singled out three great pioneers: Benjamin Rush, who made groping efforts to raise the study and treatment of mental disease to a scientific level; Dorothea Lynde Dix, who helped provide humane treatment for the afflicted through her crusade to place them in hospitals for special care and treatment; and Clifford Beers, "who brought about a synthesis of scientific and humanitarian reform in a single, organized mental hygiene movement" (p. 518).

Dorothea Dix did indeed play a major role in bringing about the current community mental health movement. It will be recalled that Miss Dix was roused to action by her discovery in 1841 of neglected insane patients in jails and poor houses. In many places, this was the mode of community care for the mentally ill, although a small number of mental hospitals did exist. Miss Dix's indomitable campaign on behalf of the mentally ill bore fruit in the form of 32 additional state hospitals. Unfortunately, they did not continue to function as the small therapeutic rural institutions that she had originally envisioned.

As population increased in the United States, increasing numbers of mentally ill people entered the mental hospitals and many stayed indefinitely. New institutions were founded as older ones overflowed. In 1866, the new 1,500 bed Willard State Hospital in New York opened solely for chronic patients, but in time all state hospitals accepted both newly ill and chronic mental patients. Bockhoven has related the subsequent history of mental hospitals which gradually grew larger (Pilgrim State Hospital, New York, housed 12,000 patients in 1955), were more crowded, and were understaffed [5].

To compound the plight of the mentally ill stuffed into asylums during the last quarter of the nineteenth century and the first quarter of the twentieth, scientific medicine had little to offer to psychiatrists. The brilliant neuropathological discoveries of the latter nineteenth century shed little light on causes of mental illness. Noguchi's discovery of the treponema in 1913, and Goldberger's finding of the etiology of pellagra dementia in 1914 gave some encouragement. Kraepelin's nosology with its gloomy prognosis of dementia praecox was refuted by Bleuler in 1911, who thought improvement of chronic states was always possible. Nor did Freud's new theories offer much to psychotic patients who Freud believed were not amenable to treatment by his new method of psychoanalysis. By contrast, advances in bacteriology and immunology were broadening the practice of public health and leading to control and prevention of many infectious diseases.

Public attitudes, based largely on ignorance of the nature of mental illness, had not changed much during the span of centuries. Mental illness was viewed as a disgrace to families in which it occurred, and the mentally ill were to be hidden from sight in their own homes or by relegation to the distant state hospital. A ray of light was shed in 1908 when Clifford Beers published *The Mind That Found Itself*, the story of his recurrent manic depressive illness and his brutal treatment in a state hospital. Beers's continuing efforts to improve the treatment of the mentally ill roused the interest of both public and psychiatric figures. The National Committee for Mental Hygiene was organized in 1909 and still continues as the National Association for Mental Health, to inform and educate Americans about mental health and illness and to improve services for the mentally ill.

Until the 1930s, few changes and innovations had occurred in the treatment of the mentally ill. The small number of psychiatrists worked mainly in the custodial state hospitals, which many people entered and relatively few left. The average rate of recovery in 1944 was 18 percent while an additional 31 percent were discharged as improved [6]. Patients with dementia praecox who died in American state mental hospitals in 1944 showed a median hospital stay of almost 15 years.

The introduction of somatic therapies gave rise to new hope. In 1933, Sakel in Vienna reported favorable results in treating schizophrenia with insulin coma therapy. The Italians Cerletti and Bini applied electroconvulsive treatment in 1933, and in 1935 Von Meduna, a Hungarian, used metrazol to induce convulsions. Both insulin and metrazol treatment have been largely abandoned, but ECT is still used to treat severe depressions. Since 1955, psychopharmacology has been the main somatic treatment in use and is credited as a major factor in the decrease of mental hospital populations thereby enabling current therapeutic approaches.

The first outpatient clinic opened at the Pennsylvania Hospital in Philadelphia in 1885, soon followed by another at the Warren (Pennsylvania) State Hospital. Similar clinics were opened in Boston and elsewhere. Child guidance clinics were first sponsored by the National Committee for Mental Hygiene in 1922, with the aim of preventing the mental ills and maladjustments of adulthood. A survey in 1946 revealed 285 children's clinics, together with 350 clinics serving both children and adults [7].

WORLD WAR II AND PSYCHIATRY THEREAFTER

The War marked a turning point in American psychiatry. The draft had disqualified more than a million young men for neuropsychiatric reasons. Large numbers of professionals and other workers were exposed to psychiatric disorders during military service. Their interest led them to enter training after the war, swelling the numbers of mental health personnel. The war expanded psychiatry's previous concern with psychoses and neuroses to include personality disorders, stress reactions, situational maladjustments, and deviant behavior. Research produced new information on leadership and the behavior of groups in various settings.

After the War, the new training programs under the V.A. and later NIMH, grew. The numbers of mental health professionals increased, particularly psychiatrists in private practice who needed hospital beds for their patients. Psychiatric units and beds in community general hospitals increased. Also after the war, public interest centered upon the sorry situation of the public mental hospitals which the war had further depleted of their scarce personnel. Deutsch exposed the dreadful conditions under which patients were living in mental hospitals, as did Gorman [8, 9]. Greenblatt, Brown, and York compared treatment and outcome in a large State mental hospital, a small state university affiliated psychopathic institute and a V.A. hospital, which showed the poorest level of patient care in the large state hospital [10].

Public outcry against shameful state hospital conditions found professional support. The First Mental Hospital Institute, sponsored by the American Psychiatric Association in Philadelphia in 1949, was attended by 190 hospital superintendents and others who related their individual horror stories of firetrap patient buildings and budgets too small to hire trained staff [11].

Most important, the postwar period produced research studies to show the noxious effects of institutional custodial care. Goffman described vividly the characteristics of total institutions and the mold into which inmates were fitted [12]. Belknap said in his book describing a southern state hospital, "Before we can expect substantial progress in our treatment of mental illness in the country, the peculiar problems posed by the social organization of the state mental hospital must be faced and solved" [13, p. XII). He described how the organization of the state hospital imposes severe limitations on the effectiveness of staff in their work with patients.

Caudill studied a small university-based mental hospital, concluding also that a psychiatric hospital is, indeed, a social system which affects the quality of behavior in all areas of hospital life and insulates both staff and patients from the community [14]. He says, "It is likely that the most effective use of modern knowledge in the treatment of patients is being impeded by outmoded administrative procedures and that some thorough going changes in the physical and organizational structure of psychiatric hospitals is long overdue" (p. 344). Further research on the psychiatric hospital as a social system is reported by Wessen [14].

As these sociological studies were proceeding in this country during the decade following World War II, interesting innovations were occurring in Great Britain. Maxwell Jones had pioneered in structuring a 'therapeutic community' for neurotic and other individuals which appeared useful in helping residents to change their behavior to become more functional [15]. Based on his experience, Jones proposed a new method of structuring large State hospitals by decentralizing them into small semi-autonomous units serving discrete geographical areas [16]. This approach, he said, improves communications intra and extramurally, allows closer ties between staff, patients and relatives, and outside agencies. The smaller treatment units also allow easier examination and modification of roles, role relationships, and the overall culture of the unit. All staff and patients are involved, at least in part, in treatment and administration. Following Jones's demonstration, a number of mental hospitals in Britain adopted the therapeutic community approach, particularly those hospitals which had unlocked patient wards. American visitors to the British mental hospitals brought back reports of these organizational and treatment innovations and, in some places, attempted to replicate these methods in American mental hospitals and psychiatric wards of general hospitals [17, 18, 19].

Based on the exposés of shameful conditions in state hospitals, buttressed by the research studies of antitherapeutic custodial mental hospitals which showed relatively little capacity to change, supported by professional and citizen mental health related organizations, the U.S. Congress passed the Mental Health Study Act in 1955, which provided funds for a nationwide study of mental health needs and resources. Six years and ten books later, the Joint Commission on Mental Illness and Health, an organization sponsored by 36 organizations, delivered its report to President Kennedy, the Congress, and the public [20]. The report recommended pursuit of new knowledge through research, better use of present knowledge and experience by training manpower, making available emergency psychiatric care, providing intensive treatment of acutely ill mental patients in clinics, general and mental hospitals, expanding the number of outpatient clinics, and establishing general hospital psychiatric units. The report urged that smaller state hospitals with 1,000 beds or less in suitable locations be converted into intensive treatment centers and that state hospitals with more than 1,000 beds become centers for long term care of physically and mentally ill people. The report stressed after-care and rehabilitation services and encouraged day and night hospitals. The Commission proposed that the cost of the program be shared by federal, state, and local governments.

One particular recommendation stands out: "Make reasonable efforts to operate open mental hospitals as mental health centers, i.e., as part of an integrated community service with emphasis on outpatient and aftercare facilities as well as inpatient services" (p. XXII). Also, "our proposal would encourage local responsibility of a degree that has not existed since the state hospital system was founded" (p. XXIII). Other recommendations were for changes in commitment laws to foster voluntary admissions, to change state laws to make treatment as well as custody a requirement in mental hospitalization, and to differentiate between the need for treatment and the need for institutionalization and to provide the former without the latter when so indicated.

The aftermath of the Joint Commission report is now history, within our memory. The National Institute of Mental Health was responsible on the federal level for providing guidance and direction to implementation of the report. The President appointed a Cabinet level committee of the Secretaries of HEW and Labor, the Administrator of the VA, and the Director of the Bureau of the Budget to prepare recommendations. On February 7, 1963, President Kennedy sent a message to Congress on mental illness and mental retardation in which he proposed a "bold new approach" through establishment of community mental health centers, while helping state mental hospitals to improve their treatment programs.

In 1963, Congress passed the Community Mental Health Centers Act. The legislation has since been amended seven times, each time broadening its scope and extending new or additional coverage to various groups including poor people and those with alcohol and drug problems. Each amendment was supported by public and professional groups. Each amendment sought to incorporate new scientific theories and findings and to utilize increased public understanding and knowledge.

Looking back, we can see how community mental health programs rose out of the bankruptcy of the state hospitals of 1946. It took 17 years following the preoccupation with World War II, to bring together the facts and public support to obtain national legislation. It is of interest that in this country efforts to improve mental health services were based on a new approach, rather than building on the existing mental hospital care system as was done in Great Britain. President Kennedy's 1963 message stressed a need to bring together all resources in a geographic area including state hospitals, and the latter were not excluded as applicants for the federal mental health center grants.

Mental hospital statistics showed little change during the decade following World War II except that both admissions and resident populations increased. Within that ten-year period, few improvements were noted in mental hospital treatment programs. It is interesting to speculate what might have happened if chlorpromazine had been available in 1945, rather than in 1955 when the work of the Joint Commission sent new thrusts underway.

Time and technology have moved swiftly. Today, thirteen years after inception of the national community mental health center program, we may examine the premises on which it is based and see if they still hold true. We will use the mental health centers program as the operational arm of community mental health practice, since a considerable body of data is available for examination.

BASIC PREMISES OF THE CMHC

The objectives set forth in the Centers Act of 1963 and its legislative history, included the provisions that community-based services should be available and accessible to all residents of designated geographic areas at all times with continuity of care, with preventive practices utilized where possible, and with continuing program evaluation. Each objective is further defined in regulations and policy.

"Comprehensive" was defined by regulation to mean at least five elements of service: inpatient, outpatient, emergency, partial hospitalization, plus consultation and education. The 1975 legislation has added seven additional elements required for eligibility for federal support, namely: services to the aged, children, transitional living facilities, followup for those leaving hospitals, screening for those who are at risk of state hospitalization, and services for people with alcohol and drug problems if such services are not otherwise available.

"Accessible" includes geographic, economic, temporal, and cultural accessibility. For instance, the new Act requires bilingual staff as needed to serve non-English speaking clientele. "Available" also means 24-hour daily service. "Continuity of care" means arrangements to provide ongoing care and service within one or more agencies according to client needs and with staff responsibility fixed for each client.

Preventive services are to be provided within available knowledge and through consultation and education programs to community care-giving agencies and to the public at large. (Preventive practices in public health are often provided through other agencies such as education, housing, and sanitation departments.) "Program evaluation" includes arrangements for continuing access to the community's assessment of mental health needs, explicit statements of program priorities, and methods to assess quality of care, client and patient progress, and outcome.

The objectives and requirements listed above were based on practical experience and research findings available twelve years ago and brought up to date since. The new world of psychopharmacology, which opened up in 1955, made community-based treatment possible for almost all patients. Only a small number require longer term or more intensive care than is available in fully functioning CMHCs (CMHC reports show that 5 to 15 percent of their clientele are transferred to mental hospitals). The earlier sociological studies of hospital structure, and the experience with therapeutic communities and open settings provided a foundation for organizing community-based services (Fort Logan Mental Health Center in Denver was established in 1961).

Research grants made available by NIMH after 1957 and by other sources to demonstrate improved treatment methods showed that alternatives to hospitalization are possible and effective [21, 22, 23]; that emergency care and crisis intervention avert longer hospitalization and are effective in restoring functioning [24, 25]; that rehabilitation programs do help restore mentally handicapped persons through sheltered living and working arrangements [26, 27]; that followup services decrease readmissions [28, 29]; that consultation to community agencies can be useful [30]; that paraprofessionals of various kinds perform useful psychotherapeutic and other functions in appropriate settings [31, 32]; that administrative and treatment information systems are possible to install and use for program planning [33]; and that the availability of adequate community services decreases state hospital admissions [34, 35, 35, 37]. A great deal of knowledge and experience is available, and not all of it is being used widely enough. Utilization of research findings and the characteristic time lag in putting them into operation remains an impediment to more effective community mental health programs.

CITIZEN PARTICIPATION

The rationale for community mental health must include consideration of "consumerism" or citizen participation. The Civil Rights movement of the 1960s helped to lay the groundwork for this development.

The social programs of the Kennedy era fostered the participation of citizens in programs designed to help them help themselves. The poverty programs operated locally by elected citizen boards are an example. Social science research provides a theoretical framework for the notion that behavior change is influenced by participant decision making [38]. Providing new roles and opportunities for decision making would raise self-esteem and increase motivation to attain socially desirable goals.

The Mental Health Centers Act of 1963, its regulations, and all its amendments until 1974 make no mention of consumer involvement. The 1975 amendments mandate that consumers comprise half of the governing boards (with the exception of publicly sponsored centers where the board may be advisory). The thrust toward consumerism began to show itself at the federal level about the mid sixties. The Public Health Amendments of 1966 mandated consumer representation on State Health Planning Councils. About the same time, NIMH policy began to foster the practice of citizen advisory boards for centers. In some places such boards had been mandated by state community mental health acts which provided for appointment of county or city governing or advisory mental health boards.

The ability of citizen boards to have a major impact on center programs has been limited. While NIMH exerted considerable pressure upon federally funded centers to appoint and use them, in many cases neither center staffs nor board members were knowledgeable about board functions, roles, and responsibilities. Many centers are based in or affiliated with general community hospitals whose governing boards usually do not represent a cross section of the catchment area. There are exceptions. The Westside Mental Health Center, a corporation in San Francisco, is operated by an elected citizen board representing local citizen organizations, providers, and individual citizens, and receives the federal grants contracting for services with providers.

The 1975 center amendments, which mandate consumer representation, are in keeping with other federal legislation. PL 93—641, Health Planning and Resources Development Act of 1974, establishes health service areas throughout the country operated by consumer majority boards as the single authority to determine health needs and allocate resources. The mental health corporation, such as the Westside Center in San Francisco, embodies the concept of consumerism and has been adopted by some centers, although this promising approach is not yet a common pattern [39]. We are currently writing regulations for implementation of the new Centers legislation and trying to make the regulations flexible enough to meet nationwide circumstances.

Consumerism will continue to influence community mental health services. Schiff has recounted his experience in Chicago, and Whitaker in Denver [40, 41]. These experiences and others suggest that citizen understanding and decisions lean more toward social rather than medically defined programs. This controversy about whether community mental health programs are social programs or medical programs remains unsettled, perhaps appropriately for the present. All our center programs have both social and medical aspects. The particular mix of personnel in any one center often determines the balance. Centers situated in poverty areas where the social components of mental disorder appear important perforce devote considerable time to community organization and interagency collaboration. Centers based in community general hospitals tend to focus more on intrapsychic individual and intrafamily problems.

Although the emphasis for centers to deal with social needs was great during the late sixties, there appears to be a swing away now, a realization that mental health workers cannot solve the tremendous social problems besetting our nation and an effort is being made to refocus center programs into more narrowly defined mental health areas. Bertram S. Brown, Director of NIMH, has written, ". . . my personal and professional belief as a physician is that the primary responsibility of the CMHC staff is to treat those . . . who are sick. This belief in no way derogates the responsibility to improve the social quality of life for individuals within the CMHC's jurisdiction" [42]. He adds that while both treatment and social reform components of the CMHC program are designed to effect change, the CMHC cannot assume responsibility for the total reform of society.

LEGAL AND JUDICIAL EVENTS

Until recent years, the courts have been concerned mainly with civil commitment of allegedly mentally ill people and with issues of mental competence in relation to legal offenses. Since 1960, the courts have begun to play an increasing role in determining the nature of mental health care. While the legal issues generally concern state mental hospitals, their thrust is to move the focus of care to less restrictive and better equipped community facilities.

Deutsch recounts the interesting tale of Mrs. E.P.W. Packard, who believed her husband had her committed to an Illinois State hospital in 1860 to get rid of her [43]. When she was discharged, she began a successful campaign for protection of allegedly insane persons. Her efforts resulted in new commitment laws being enacted in Illinois, Massachusetts, and Iowa, and indirectly affected lunacy legislation in other states.

Until about 1950, admissions to public mental hospitals were mainly through court commitment. The number has gradually declined. In 1972, 42 percent of admissions to public mental hospitals were involuntary. Much state legislation has been passed in the last ten years revising state commitment laws. The Lanterman-Petris-Short Act in California (1968) requires that prospective admissions to state hospitals must first be screened and treated in local facilities. The Baker Act in Florida (1971) abolishes indefinite commitment, requiring that all involuntary patients may be retained for a period not to exceed six months, following which another hearing must be held. New York state law requires that the prospective patient must be fully informed of his rights and be provided legal counsel.

Danger to self and others is increasingly accepted as the only legitimate criterion for involuntary commitment. Nine states and the District of Columbia currently restrict commitment to dangerous patients [44]. In Massachusetts, evidence of dangerous behavior must be presented at a hearing. Some states have abolished indefinite commitment and require periodic rehearings. Recently, legal argument has been heard to the effect that confinement should not be used if alternative treatment outside the institution is possible and preferable. This is the crux of a case decided against Saint Elizabeth's Hospital in Washington, D.C. [45]. Stone notes that the "least restrictive alternative" approach, although it embodies the community mental health model, causes concern to clinicians practicing in the community. Treatment is a quid pro quo for loss of liberty. He adds that the thrust of the Saint Elizabeth's lawsuit is to require that treatment and care be provided outside the hospital walls [46].

The right to treatment issue has major significance. *Rouse* vs. *Cameron* was the first major legal decision to deal with this issue [47]. The court decision asked for a bonafide effort to provide patients with an individualized treatment program and periodic evaluation, and denied that insufficient resources was an adequate justification for failure to provide treatment. *Wyatt* v. *Stickney* (now *Wyatt* v. *Alderholt*) affirmed the constitutional right to treatment for those mentally disordered persons who are involuntarily civilly committed [48, 49]. In *Burnham* v. *Georgia*, this same right was denied [50]. The *Wyatt* v. *Stickney* case resulted in the court setting standards for facilities and a detailed program for improving conditions for patient care at the Bryce State Hospital in Tuscaloosa, Alabama.

The cases mentioned above were decided by lower courts, but in *O'Connor* v. *Donaldson*, the Supreme Court (in June 1975) said that a mental patient not dangerous to himself or others and who is not getting treatment, has a constitutional right to be discharged from custodial care if he can survive safely in freedom [51]. Other legal decisions have been taken to safeguard patient rights to freedom, to treatment, to confidentiality of their records, to deny the administration of medication or somatic therapies. State laws are incorporating these decisions. Montana passed a new mental health code in 1975 (Senate Bill #377, Chapter #466, Montana Session Laws of 1975) incorporating a patient Bill of Rights in detail—i.e., every patient must have an individualized treatment plan.

In general, these judicial holdings are consistent with community mental health philosophy and practice. The federal strategy which promotes development of CMHCs reduces reliance on state institutions, creates a range of alternative treatment modes, focuses on the specific needs of high risk groups, is in tune with the court decrees. Ironically, however, by focusing on institutional failures and demanding instant remedy, the judiciary may be inadvertently pumping scarce resources into asylums rather than into community alternatives.

SOME UNRESOLVED ISSUES

The medical versus the social basis for mental health center operations has not been resolved. Nor does a solution readily appear. Our experience suggests that the issue is best decided by the local community to be served. It is likely that resolution may come, at least in part, through decisions of third-party payors.

An important issue now confronting us is the provision of support services to thousands of mentally handicapped people living in communities, many of whom are ex-state hospital patients. We do not know their numbers, but the resident patient population in public mental hospitals is close to 350,000 fewer than in 1955, down to something more than 200,000 patients. In addition, approximately 400,000 patients each year have been admitted to and discharged since then from public mental hospitals. Many of these people have returned to their families, some are in sheltered living arrangements, many are living alone in back rooms. The GAO has just completed a study of deinstitutionalization for Congress. The gaps in followup care have been carefully documented. Much work must be done at federal, regional, state, and local levels to build the structures a community support system requires. Our Division of Mental Health Service Programs is actively engaged in developing the needed concepts, elements and strategies to deal with this serious problem.

The issue of quality of care is a salient one at present for all of medicine. The Social Security amendments of 1972 mandating PSRO activities in hospitals and health facilities to certify quality care in order to receive federal payment under Medicare and Medicaid, will also apply to mental health centers. The new center legislation requires that utilization and peer review be instituted in all funded centers. The American Psychiatric Association and other groups have issued criteria and guidelines, but the implementation of procedures is still rudimentary in most places. Zusman has pointed out the difficulties [52]. We are still engaged in research to produce tools with which to measure or even to determine the elements in quality care. The goal attainment scaling method is a promising approach to judging outcome [53].

VIEWPOINT IN RETROSPECT

We have watched the development of a community mental health approach for over 20 years, if we consider its inception with the start of the work of the Joint Commission on Mental Illness and Health. We are struck by the prescience of the men and women who guided the Commission's work and the implementation of the recommendations. How could they foresee the Civil Rights movement of the sixties, the judicial decisions and state mental health codes of the seventies, and shape the mental health center movement accordingly? The structure and program of the centers can meet the current demands of society and the law. Perhaps the reciprocal view can also be taken. The centers experience helped shape the consumer movement and the judicial decisions.

Looking back, it does seem that the decision to branch off independently and not build on the existing state hospital system was appropriate. Some state hospitals have become truly therapeutic short-stay institutions, but too many still do not have the resources or the power to move in that direction. Conversely, it would not have been possible to build on an entirely private system of care. Resources have not been and are not available, and solo practice cannot provide a comprehensive range of services. Perhaps group practice might have worked out, but financing of private medical care is still unresolved in this country. We view the CMHC as one part of a pluralistic system of mental health care, and hope that "current and necessary preoccupation with law, politics, economics and administration does not drown the dream of better care for all people" [54, p. 13].

VIEWPOINT IN PROSPECT

A new problem looms: how do we reconcile the strength and values of the community mental health concept with the current reality of political, economic, and bureaucratic catastrophe? This is a dark hour for dreams, when Congress and the Executive are farther apart than ever with respect to CMHC budget and federal role; when Commissioners are better known as defendants in law suits than as architects of new programs; when vacancies in leadership positions at all levels of health (and mental health) administration are commonplace. To understand this phenomenon and to maintain enthusiasm for and dedication to the still valid principles and values of community mental health, we suggest a broad view of civilization which borrows some insights from both Aristotle's *Poetics*, with his views on tragedy, and Erikson's thoughts on integrity [55, 56].

We seem to be at the end of an epoch. Just as the Classic Age in Greece, the Dark Ages, and the Elizabethan Era closed and were replaced, this Age of Expansion is ending. It has not been an age without achievements. We have seen dramatic scientific advances, startling insights into human behavior, and long overdue shifts in values and power with respect to sex and race. A predominant characteristic of this epoch has been acceleration in all things. But as the current themes dissipate, we can expect some of the inevitable feelings of loss, frustration, anger, and confusion that inevitably precede acceptance of an end. In poetic tragedy, this moment displays something noble, larger than life, revealing a cosmic order, and the significance of human kind; and the result is exultation, not despair.

In Erikson's view, the final crisis, for which we prepare throughout life, is a realization or a failure to realize that life is an integrated whole; that it could not and should not have been significantly different. The feeling tone one associates with the successful realization may not be as dramatic as Greek tragedy, but nevertheless it is a proud and positive emotion. Furthermore, integrity comes on the heels of generativity. The individual has created posterity and created for posterity.

In these concepts, millenia apart, are reasons enough for fierce dedication to the dreams of a dying era. For the principles of community mental health are noble. And the demonstrated ability of people in neighborhoods to define complicated issues and launch comprehensive programs is a template for some future form of social interdependence which will work in the epoch that replaces this one.

SUMMARY

The rationale for community mental health stems from the attitudes of society. The social ethos at any given time has always determined the fate and treatment of mentally ill, emotionally troubled, and behaviorally deviant people. Through political process, social attitudes are translated into laws which are clarified through judicial process. Medical, biologic, and social sciences contribute knowledge that influence social values, the political process, and judicial decisions. Community mental health in 1976 is a reflection of these processes at this moment in time.

Should this entire age of western civilization close and be replaced by some new social order, as we believe it inevitably will, the principles of community mental health shall survive that epochal metamorphosis and shall provide a foundation for some new arrangements whereby individuals in workable groups define human problems and discover solutions.

> We will grieve not, rather find
> Strength in what remains behind;
> In the primal sympathy
> Which having been must ever be;
> In the soothing thoughts that spring
> Out of human suffering;
> In the faith that looks through death,
> In the years that bring the philosophic mind.
> —William Wordsworth,
> *Ode: Intimations of Immortality*

A Critical Appraisal of
Community Health Services

Stanley F. Yolles

I begin my contribution to this discussion with a statement about cats. *All* cats are grey in the dark. Grimalkin is a grey cat. Therefore, he is in the dark. This is a syllogism, an example of deductive reasoning which by definition may be subtle, tricky, or specious. I would suggest to you that much of the criticism of the community mental health centers program is syllogistic—which is a polite way of saying that it is less than complete.

In any field, some criticism is ignorant, some is self-serving, and some is sound. In the field of community mental health, a great deal of criticism comes from nonsense rather than common sense and demonstrates everything from faulty logic to destructive intent. It has become fashionable in some circles to say that community mental health centers have failed. Those who cry "failure" give (at best) piecemeal evidence; and *no one* to my knowledge has come up with anything approaching an alternative plan for mental health services adaptable to the mental health needs of an entire population or segment thereof.

I am, therefore, exceedingly pleased to have this opportunity to discuss the *rationale* from which the comprehensive community mental health services program has been and continues to be developed. In the name of sweet reason, I shall attempt to limit myself to the rationale by which a concept was translated into an operational system of human services. Because of the limited time available for this discussion, I will have little to say about "great expectations," Dickensian, Johnsonian, or otherwise. I will have a little more to say about how performance has not—as yet—fulfilled the potential for *maximum* performance, even though I expect to demonstrate that the quality of the program's performance is high enough to support my belief that (if we were to start all over again) we would—to a large extent—set the program up in the same way.

I begin with a question: Why is it, at a time when cynicism is so great that people are surprised if *anything* works well (from a TV set to a college curriculum), that community mental health programs are faulted because they have not done away with all mental illness in ten years? The answer comes in part from that fact that both those people old enough to know have forgotten what they are talking about, and those too young to have been present at the creation and who (while steeped in the nostalgia of "The Great Gatsby" or "The Sting"), show little interest when professionals in psychiatry and the behavioral sciences try to tell them how things were before.

Before what? Well, let's return briefly to how things were when Congress provided the funds in 1955 under the Mental Health Study Act to establish the National Commission on Mental Illness and Health and six years later when the report was published. The Joint Commission received a mandate from Congress to survey the resources and to make recommendations for combatting mental illness in the United States. This had *never before* been attempted on a national basis. Even the states appeared content to perpetuate the moribund and self-protective system in which mental patients were sequestered in state hospitals, where care was a euphemism provided in large part through "protective detention" rather than treatment.

This system had become so rigid that the task of the Joint Commission (even in trying to find out what was actually happening in these hospitals) was as difficult as trying to carve Mount Rushmore with an ice pick. Others had also tried—notably, S. Weir Mitchell, in an address before the Fiftieth Annual Meeting of the American Medico-Psychological Association in *1894*. Following the Civil War, Mitchell's medical interest became concentrated on disorders of the nervous system. He is generally regarded as the father of American neurology. In accepting this speaking engagement, Mitchell warned his audience, who were medical superintendents of "American institutions for the Insane," that he would "speak boldly and with no regard to persons."

You can find the entire address in *Classics of American Psychiatry*, which was published in 1975 by W.H. Green in St. Louis. Here are a few of Mitchell's comments, as he stood before the men who controlled the fate of every individual patient within those hospitals:

> It is the system which is most to blame, (but) my fear is that some of
> you would not change your organization if you could. . . . You live alone,
> uncriticized, unquestioned, out of the healthy conflicts and honest rivalries

which keep us up to the mark of the fullest possible competence. The whole system has been let to harden into organized shapes which are difficult to reform.

You ought not to live and sleep in your hospitals at all; you ought to be in contact with the world of sane men, having consultations outside, seeing us and our societies. A good deal of this can never be had in your hospitals, for incredible folly has put most of them remote from cities. . . .

I may be wrong as to some men and some hospitals, but fifty years hence, another will possibly stand in my place and tell your history, and to him and the beautiful wisdom of time, I leave it to be declared whether I was right or wrong.

As the Joint Commission reported, some sixty years later, Mitchell had *not* been wrong. The Commission published its final report *Action for Mental Health* in 1961. Its findings established the foundations upon which the national mental health program continues to be developed.

In February 1963, for the first time in the nation's history, a President of the United States—John F. Kennedy—sent a message on mental illness to the Congress, because, as he said, "the problem is of such critical size and tragic impact and the susceptibility to public action is deserving of a wholly new national approach."

Terming results to improve conditions in state hospitals "too often dismal," President Kennedy had this to say to the Congress:

> Some States have at times been forced to crowd five, ten, or even fifteen thousand people into one large understaffed institution. The following statistics are illustrative:
>
> Nearly one-fifth of the 279 State mental institutions are fire and health hazards; three-fourths of them were opened prior to World War I.
>
> Nearly half of the 530,000 patients in our State mental hospitals are in institutions with over 3,000 patients.

I would add parenthetically here that at the time, eighteen hospitals housed 5,000 or more patients and an occasional hospital had a patient load of close to 20,000.

> President Kennedy continued by pointing out that: . . . many of these institutions have less than half the professional staff required—with less than one psychiatrist for every 360 patients. . . . Forty-five percent of their inmates have been hospitalized continuously for ten years or more.

If one looks further into the data on which President Kennedy based his message to Congress, the record becomes far worse than dismal. It was a dreadful situation. For example, only 28 percent of the state mental hospitals (in 1961) had been able to meet the criteria for accreditation by the Joint Commission on Accreditation. Even worse, the rate of accreditation had declined. The proportion of all public mental hospitals rated as "nonacceptable" had risen from 14 percent in 1950 to 28 percent in 1961. Also in 1961, over one-third of the mental hospitals in the United States were more than 75 years old and many of the original buildings are still in use. (Indeed, some of them are still in use in 1977.)

These examples are illustrative of many other findings that when assembled and published forced superintendents of state mental hospital systems to come out of their isolation wards and face the facts— the facts that could no longer be ignored:

As the population of the United States increased, so did the mental hospital population. Even with the initial use of psychotropic drugs, most patients faced a lifetime of institutional custody. Projections of patient population showed clearly that, unless there was a radical change in the system of care and treatment of the mentally ill, the cost of mental illness throughout the United States would skyrocket. More patients would bring about more hospital construction, higher operating budgets, and continuation of a situation which the public and the health professions had begun to realize was insupportable.

THE CMHC PROGRAM

The Community Mental Health Centers Act of 1963, with its statement of federal support, provided the first opportunity to initiate a new approach to the care and treatment of the mentally ill on a national scope. I think it pertinent to quote the 1963 definition: "A comprehensive community mental health center is a multi-service community facility designed to provide preventive services, early diagnosis and treatment of mental disorders, both on an inpatient and outpatient basis, and to serve as a locus for the after-care of discharged hospital patients."

The National Institute of Mental Health was charged with the responsibility to implement the statute. Its fundamental concept (based on the above definition) called for a service program located in local communities, rather than in isolated custodial institutions. The first and basic objective of the Community Mental Health Centers program, therefore, was to *decrease* the utilization of state mental hospitals. This was not the *only* objective, but it was certainly first on the list and the rationale for the program developed from that basic goal.

I have not been assigned the task of presenting a 1976 progress report; but I would like to point out that in terms of this objective, the community mental health centers program has not failed. Accumulating evidence, nationwide, indicates that the rate of hospital population has declined as mental health centers come into operation.

In 1967 there were more than 426,000 patients resident in state hospitals across the country. At the end of 1972, the number had declined to 276,000—a drop of 150,000, or 35 percent in just five years. It is also clear that those areas of the country covered by mental health centers are doing much better than those not covered. In areas where CMHCs have been open for three years or more, the probability that a person will be resident in a state hospital is only 70 percent of the national average. In Kentucky, where mental health centers are available to the entire population, the resident state hospital population has dropped by nearly 50 percent. Other data indicate that the patients' length of stay in state mental hospitals is coming down. There are various reasons for this, but a 1972 study of matched areas indicated that a decline in length of hospital stay, longer than one year, was six times greater in an area served by a community mental health center than in an area without one.

These changes have not come about solely because of the physical presence of the five to six hundred community mental health centers now in operation across the country. Something else has been happening. Saul Feldman put it succinctly, writing in 1974 in the *International Journal of Mental Health*:

> There has been a discernible change in the mental health *Zeitgeist*, stimulated in good measure by the ideology of the community mental health centers program. We have been experiencing our own cultural revolution in mental health and our values are changing as a result.
>
> Care in the community, alternatives to hospitalization, briefer stays when hospitalization does become necessary, and more recognition of the iatrogenic effects of institutionalization are now almost taken for granted. *This was not so ten years ago.* Our treatment services are changing, not because our patients are really any different, but because *we* are. These are extremely important changes, in which the community mental health center program has played an intangible but central role.

I would supplement this statement by pointing out that some of the program influence stems from tangible as well as intangible program characteristics, and that they were consciously designed as program components from the first strategy meetings in which the rationale for a program was set forth in regulations and guidelines for administration of the statute.

RATIONALE AND REGULATIONS

I can review, outline, delineate, protect, defend, and explain every step in the rationale from which the original regulations governing the administration of the Community Mental Health Act were evolved. But not in this space. Therefore, I shall be indicative, rather than comprehensive, in my comment.

Community psychiatry is based on the adaptation of public health practice to mental health service. Its objective is to provide high quality care to population groups, or communities. In 1963, no one had defined the composition of "a community" in these terms. For the community mental health centers program, a community was defined primarily in terms of *numbers of people* for whom services are to be provided. The rationale for this was, above all else, to make sure that CMHC Centers would not—like the state mental hospitals —become overcrowded, overwhelmed, unresponsive administrative units. From this point of view, the "catchment area" concept originated and has become operational. Criticism of this plan has really become outmoded. Inequities have been and are negotiated and the original purpose of the fiat has been proved viable.

In relation to the needs of patients, rather than the perceived needs of administrators, the CMHC program established a requirement for continuity of care for each patient-client. It has been some time since I have heard any responsible citizen argue against the concept of "continuity of care," for even though the difficulties of providing for it are sometimes great, the means to achieve it—given adequate resources—are now accepted.

In the realm of administration, acceptance of the concept has increased; ability to deliver still lags behind knowledge. In setting up a service system, the CMHC designers pioneered in demonstrating the feasibility of providing treatment for an individual by assembling service units under one administrative umbrella. As it turns out, what this requires is the establishment under law of administrative agreements among agencies prepared to provide stated kinds of service. This idea is now old hat throughout the entire health industry; it was very "new hat" in 1963.

Much of the administrative hassle stemmed from the argument— deeply felt and often expressed indirectly—about who was to run the show. This has brought forth many kinds of subterfuge. What it boils down to is a combination of professional protective coloration, rejection of change, and refusal to make interdisciplinary cooperation something more than a shibboleth or a dirty word. Here again, the failures come from sloth and bad faith, as well as from the very real difficulties in making interdisciplinary concepts work on a daily and yearly basis. Some who have tried it like it; others do not. So be it. If the public demands it I would predict that the interdisciplines will provide it or perish. And others—courts, lawyers, consumers, politicians—will indeed "run" the psychiatric show, rather than the mental health professionals.

Again, I think that the bricks and mortar syndrome as a criticism has been put to rest within the mausoleum of yesterday. Proponents of the Community Mental Health Centers Act, in attempting to secure federal support for mental health services, had to approach Congress on tiptoe. This is almost unbelievable for the current generation of mental health trainees in all disciplines. However, it was necessary to "tease" Congress into providing *some* money to fund the construction of *some* buildings. But before applicants could get the money (unlike Hill-Burton funding) under the Community Mental Health Centers Act, the programmatic elements had to be approved; and there were more than a few innovations. However, the original statute was limited. This was true not because of a lack of perception on the part of the proponents of community mental health; it was simply a realization that the camel's nose could get under the tent—publicly— that far and no farther at that time.

The degree of congressional acceptance was demonstrated conclusively when Congress refused, on the first go-round, to approve federal support for payment of staff salaries in community mental health centers. This was corrected in the 1965 Amendments, when staffing funds, and a formula for continuation of staffing funds, became part of the statute. But here again the rationale was not at fault; it was simply unacceptable to the congressional thinking of that day.

Sadly, that time lag in the provision of federal aid to staffing resulted in the operational inability of the National Institute of Mental Health to monitor performance of the new Centers adequately; nor could the NIMH require an evaluation of performance from staffs over which the NIMH had no fiduciary control. Staffing grant procedures continue to be refined. As this progression continues, minitoring of performance should improve.

In looking back to the source of today's critiques of the CMHC program, any objective analyst must not forget that, after a century-and-a-half of less than benign neglect of the mentally ill, a federal government agency was working with state and local public officials, with a part of the medical profession unaccustomed to cooperating with anybody (to put it mildly), and with citizen champions of the mentally ill to structure a treatment and service program that would work from Mississippi to Montana.

So, there were criticisms about the regulation that required mental health center administration to provide five essential services under that continuity-of-care umbrella. Generally, psychiatry as a profession accepted the idea that a continuity of kinds and degrees of service should be available to a patient, ranging from inpatient services to after-care. The major battle was drawn over timing. In 1963, NIMH required all qualifying CMHCs to provide the range of five services: inpatient, outpatient, emergency, partial hospitalization, and consultation and education. The rationale, born of experience, was both time and patient oriented. If CMHCs were allowed to add services step by step, some of them would never add them, but merely continue to provide whatever services they were able to mount in order to receive federal support.

I do not remember anyone who argued that such a service range would be anything but beneficial for patients. But I do remember a great deal of anguish about timing. This conflict is still with us. The 1975 Amendments to the Centers Act provide for a two-year lead time before new mental health centers are required to provide all essential services. In my opinion, this is a regrettable recession from the original service requirement. On balance, however, the acceptance of a potential for increased CMHC services has widened. In the Amendments of 1970 as well as those of 1975, the Community Mental Health Act now provides (more in verbiage than in dollars) for federal support of additional services in alcoholism, drug abuse, children's services, services for the elderly—as well as for an increasingly specific range of rehabilitative services, sheltered work situations, half-way houses, job-training programs, and others. Most, if not all of these service concepts, however, stem from a concern for those individuals who are already mentally ill or emotionally disturbed.

At the other end of the spectrum, the rationale for the national mental health program also included (as an essential service) the establishment of a consultation and education service, known as C and E. C and E was designed to achieve several things. It was seen first as a means to develop preventive mental health services in a community by requiring the CMHC staffs to initiate communitywide exchange on a routine basis with the staffs of all relevant community agencies. In so doing, it would operate to break down professional isolation and agency barriers to the benefit of the staffs, the clients, and the taxpayers.

C and E has not developed as effectively as had been planned. The idea was new; in fact, this was the first time in any federal health statute were a preventive service had been declared to be mandatory. In the 1975 Amendments, provision is made to provide for a separate system of grants, specifically available to consultation and education programs in community mental health centers. If and when the requisite funding is provided, the dollar incentive should stimulate the preventive aspects of the entire CMHC program.

This reminds me of another area in which the rationale behind the plan was correct, but where implementation has been inadequate. It was apparent early on that there would be a residual 15 percent or so of mental patients who cannot be treated and cared for effectively in a community setting, but who are not sick enough to need 24-hour hospitalization. For them, a humane and helpful residential treatment environment must be evolved. They must not be left to die in the back wards of state mental hospitals. We know now how to provide a better fate for them; and utilization of this knowledge in their behalf should have a major priority among mental health professionals and those who can provide the funding and other resources necessary.

Until now I have been summarizing the critical debates which by and large were conducted in a professional and reasonable manner by the proponents and adversaries of each part of the community mental health centers program. But in some other areas, criticism has become highly emotional and fact gives way to fantasy. One of these critical areas is a can of worms that has become known as "the medical model" debate.

One group claims that community mental health centers should be directed by a psychiatrist (aided by psychologists, nurses, and social workers) and should limit their services to the treatment of those who are already mentally ill. Within this group there is a division about what kinds of mental illness should be treated and on what priority. Some opt for first priority for the psychotic, and others would give priority to neuroses and some behavioral dysfunctions. This group, apparently, will resist to the death any broadening of the range of services.

In direct opposition are those who demand that community mental health center staffs address themselves to righting the social and economic wrongs of their neighborhood environments. They insist (sometimes violently) that anything from landlord boycotts to ethnic and racial protests come under the responsiblity of the mental health center to promote the mental health of the population. As an offshoot of this conflict, there are those who claim that paraprofessionals, indigenous personnel, ex-drug addicts, and volunteers should control the resources, the staffs, and the set of the program.

It has been my experience that none of the advocates, of any point of view, in this debate has presented a definitive rationale. Somewhat wearily, but quite emphatically, I would remind you that the rationale for both administration and programming has from its inception allowed for a flexible range of services. Those who drew up the guidelines were very much aware of the traditional inflexibilities and/or the radical experimentation demanded by various persons in various parts of the country. If one looks dispassionately at the regulations and guidelines, it is obvious that each community mental health center, each state, and each city or county has a great opportunity to make of each program what they will—based on a consensus of the perceived needs of each catchment area.

Certainly, the rationale was based on what I pointed out at the outset as an overriding need to provide the bulk of treatment of the mentally ill outside state mental hospitals. Beyond that—and with a minimum of restrictions—each community mental health center has been given the opportunity for independent action. Some of the events that have occurred because of this ferment have been beneficial in causing adversaries to learn the value of cooperation and compromise. I would point out, however, that the debate has opened the doors to others—consumer groups, the legal bar, the courts, the legislators, and the executive branch of the federal government—who are now making legislative, judicial, and budgetary decisions that will severely limit the leadership role of mental health professionals unless the professionals assume the leadership roles available.

And then there are those who make their reputations by trumpeting their belief that mental illness is a myth. Here again, the reasoning is syllogistic and in some instances professionally irresponsible. There is much more to this than a debate between conservatives and radicals. Certainly it is true that some behavior considered bizarre in one culture is acceptable in another. But that is not the point. In the past fifteen years, through technology and research investigations, knowledge of the function and dysfunction of the brain has progressed dramatically. If mental illness is indeed a myth, it is a myth that has firm bases in genetics, neuropharmacology, and neurophysiology. The knowledge about the physiologic and psychologic orders and disorders of man's psyche and soma, and the clinical means to alleviate symptoms (if not as yet to cure), make the demogoguery of the "myth-sayers" ridiculous—if it were not for the human capacity for wishful thinking.

The point I would make here is that the rationale behind the entire national mental health program was and is based on a progressive plan to support development of resources for training of personnel, for research, and for clinical and human services. At no time has this rationale been anything but global in its purpose and its approach.

In conclusion, I would again ask those who oppose the community mental health centers concept what they propose as a substitute. Would they send all the patients back to state mental hospitals? Whether they realize it or not, the public and the professionals *are* taking for granted some of the practices in mental health services that would disappear. For, although community-based care is not available to all the population, it is available widely enough so that it has generated a public expectation that more community care, not less, will become available.

To community residents who resent the so-called "dumping" of mental patients in the community, I would suggest that the "dumping" exists only because the legislatures and the communities have not provided the services necessary to maintain former mental patients *in the community*, to the mutual benefit of everyone concerned. What would they do with persons suffering from schizophrenia? Lock them up again and throw the key away? Should we ignore what we know about treatment and maintenance, while fighting our internecine battles? On the contrary, the entire mental health community has arrived at a time in which knowledge and a reasoned use thereof can bring into practice the mental health service programs that were projected in the 1960s.

If this is to occur, the entrenched interests must get out of the trenches. If they do not, they may well be digging their own graves.

Discussant: The Need
for Further Study

Alexander Leighton

I find these two papers most impressive, and I suspect that when history looks on the mental health movement it will find it to be the work of men and women with extraordinary vision and extraordinary achievement. I think that, if anything, the authors have understated the odds in the struggle. It has been more like one David against ten Goliaths. I have had the opportunity occasionally to stand close to people in government who were trying to bring about great humanitarian changes. One can only be struck by the size, the complexity, and the power of the restrictions they face. I'm grateful that I've been asked to comment, but very conscious of how easy it is to have callow temerity.

The Need to Obtain Information
The main point among the several I want to make is *the importance of having the rationale of policy and the conduct of operations serviced by information obtained through scientific processes.* I am far from maintaining that this has not occurred, but I do raise the question of whether it has occurred enough. Has it been more in words than deeds? As Dr. Yolles pointed out, sometimes intentions are on the books, but money for implementation is not authorized by Congress. Will such discrepancies continue in the future? We hear much nowadays, as Dr. Ochberg mentioned, about how we know more than we practice. This is likely, true enough, but in a number of areas in the mental health field I think we practice more than we know—sometimes far more than we know, with disastrous effects.

The work on which this paper is based was supported under National Health & Development Project #604 1042 22(48) of the Department of National Health & Welfare of Canada.

45

Let me develop a little further the historical trend we have established, and begin at an earlier time in France and England, the beginning of the nineteenth century. This was when the 'Great Mental Hospital Movement' got underway, expressing the ideas of such people as Pinel and Tuke to the effect that mental illness is curable, that environment is all important, and that mental hospitals can be created to provide that environment. It should consist of a regime that is kind but firm, building healthy minds and healthy bodies. It should contain a balance of work, exercise, and recreation; there should be music, religious services, lectures by distinguished speakers, and constant encouragement for the patients to develop wholesome thinking. They would thus become restored to their natural dignity as human beings, and to their self-confidence. The words "moral treatment" are familiar as a name for this movement, though I suspect that "moral" in those days had a broader meaning than it does today.

The world outside the hospital was considered a bad place for the mentally ill, a place that at best prevented recovery and at worst did harm. It seems likely that the model in people's minds was something like the treatment of a fracture: a broken leg is put in a cast for protection and to allow healing, and the patient is supported by good food, good general medication, and friendly care. It was thought that if the mentally ill person were brought into a hospital early enough and were separated from the evil influences of the community, he or she would be certain to recover and go back again to the world with coping abilities regained.

These views were charged with very strong feelings in Europe and America. While I am not a historian, it seems to me that they were associated with those more general humanitarian values characteristic of the first half of the nineteenth century. Thus they were part of the feeling that abolished slavery, repealed the corn laws, brought about Catholic emancipation in the United Kingdom, and the liberal revolt of 1848 in Europe. It was the age when public health came into existence, and when Virkow said that poverty was the cause of typhus, and went into the Prussian Parliament in order to fight for the poor.

The proponents of hospital environmental treatment were convinced of inevitable success, and they endeavored to sell their convictions with claims of 80 to 100 percent cure. On the basis of such expectations large sums of money were given to provide public hospitals for the mentally ill, the money coming at first from private sources and then later from the state. Yet there was very little substantiation for the effectiveness of the treatment. It was a matter of a belief that had an enormous appeal to people's convictions about what was right. The lack of scientific support was due to the inadequacy of scientific thinking at the time, and there were those who called for evidence. But the emotional conviction of rightness was too impatient and too strong. The program grew and marched on, far ahead of its data.

After mid century, however, a counter-trend set in. People began to think that the results in the hospitals were not living up to expectations, and Pliny Earle, among others, challenged the statistics of the superintendents by pointing out that the denominator they used when they claimed 80 to 100 percent recovery was the number of patients discharged, not the number of patients admitted (Grob 1973).

The hospitals had been gradually filling up through the years, like the silting bed of the Mississippi, with more and more patients who were "incurable," to use the word of the time. While ignored in the reporting of therapeutic successes, this precipitate clogged the workings of the hospitals and reduced the number of beds available for new cases, unfortunately including those who might have had a good chance of recovery if treated early. This increase in numbers of long term patients was the result of several factors such as population growth due to births and immigration from Europe, especially of European poor, who apparently had a high rate of mental illness.

Pessimism replaced the former optimism after the middle of the nineteenth century. People became alarmed about costs, especially costs of programs that did not show any demonstrable success. This concern was greatly exacerbated by the occurrence of a major economic depression in 1873, followed by another one in the 1890s. What is interesting, important, and sad is that the decline of the mental hospital movement was as lacking in factual knowledge as was its rise.

It seems to me that when mental hospitals were able to operate somewhere close to the moral treatment ideal, it is very likely that they did some good for their patients, maybe quite a lot, even if they never approached the extravagant claims of cure. Much might have been learned by systematic examination of what they actually were doing and by followup studies of what actually happened to their patients. The withdrawal, however, of interest and financial support from the mental hospitals in the latter half of the nineteenth century was as nonrational as was its rise in the first half.

The parallels with our own period are, I believe, worthy of consideration. One can argue that facts alone cannot stem popular, economic, and political forces. Indeed it may seem naive to have any such faith in the power of truth when up against aroused and headstrong opinion in the body politic. Yet, naive or not, I think facts can help, if they provide both anchor points that sooner or later have effects, and ammunition for dealing with what Dr. Yolles calls "specious arguments." Certainly without such anchor points one has nothing. The 'Great Mental Health Center Movement' has repeated the errors of the 'Great Mental Hospital Movement' by inadequate attention to the scientific evaluation of effectiveness.

Confusion of Terms

A second major suggestion I have is that there has been, and continues to be, serious error in *mistaking difficulties about the use of terms referring to mental illnesses for difficulties in recognizing the phenomena.* The confusion of terms is of course enormous, with (at the apex) the employment of "mental health" to mean mental illness. On the other hand, the behavioral phenomena that constitute mental illnesses appear as patterns, or syndromes, which are fairly consistent and which occur and recur across many different kinds of populations.

At our School of Public Health I have had much to do with physicians, psychologists, nurses, lawyers, social workers, anthropologists, and sociologists who are interested in, and sincerely dedicated to, improving mental health services. There is great difficulty convincing these highly intelligent and well trained students that there are any consistent phenomena—indeed any objective facts—known about mental illness.

It has been said at this meeting that the "lunatic fringe" ideas of the 1960s are now fading, and this may be so; but I cannot help being impressed that many of the students who come to us have closed minds. They already know that there is no such thing as mental illness, except insofar as it is caused by the prejudices of society and the misguided efforts of those psychiatrists who act as society's agents. Let me repeat that these are very intelligent, and motivated, advanced students, and it is certain that before long many will be in policy making positions of some power. If they continue to think as they do now, the results will be exceedingly serious for the mentally ill—and for society.

Those who are gathered at this meeting recognize that independent observers are able to identify the phenomena of mental illness with a reasonable degree of reliability. This is demonstrated in the work of Dohrenwend and Dohrenwend (1969) and Spitzer (1974) in New York; Kety and his colleagues (1968) with the Copenhagen data; Essen-Moller (1956) and Hagnell (1966) in Sweden; Wing, Cooper, and Sartorious (1974) in London and Geneva; and my coworkers of the Stirling County Study in Canada and Africa (D. Leighton et al., 1963 and A. Leighton et al., 1963).

While using somewhat different systems, each of these has demonstrated that is is possible to identify and classify mental illness phenomena with a high degree of interobserver reliability. Each group has found that when terms are given operational definitions, and are used consistently, independent observers are able to agree to an extent that argues strongly not only for the reality but also the frequency of the phenomena in different populations and across cultural lines. These facts should be better known, and there is need for more studies designed to serve as objective demonstrations with a view to influencing policy.

Let me be a little more specific and illustrate with a few tables. These are taken from the Stirling County Study and pertain to an outpatient clinic that we initiated in 1951 (J. Murphy and A. Leighton, 1976). The catchment area has a population of about 20,000 and virtually everyone who receives any kind of formal mental illness service, does so through the clinic. As I have mentioned, we developed our own version of a system of operational definitions and held them constant through time. Table 1—1 shows adult first admissions for two calendar years that are fifteen years apart—1952 and 1967.

The similarity in the distributions among the different categories of disorder is noteworthy. Yet between 1952 and 1967 there were several turnovers in staff, major educational campaigns about mental health occurred, a local branch of the Canadian Medical Health Association was formed, and the provincial and federal government augmented available funds. Despite all this, and other changes, it would seem that for some reason, or reasons, the population of the geographic area furnished to the clinic, at both points, consisted of essentially the same proportions of the main types of disorder. The clinic's policy was to accept everything and there was no waiting list.

Table 1—1. Primary Diagnosis of New Admission Adult Patients Seen in 1952 and 1967

	1952		1967	
	No.	%	*No.*	%
Psychosis	(18)	22	(15)	24
Psychoneurosis	(38)	47	(26)	41
Personality disorder	(10)	12	(6)	9
Brain syndrome	(9)	11	(8)	13
Other	(6)	8	(8)	13
Total	(81)	100	(63)	100

Another point of interest is that psychosis, psychoneurosis, and brain syndrome are all conditions that commonly require medication. Altogether in 1967 these amounted to some 75 percent of first admissions. Many such people needed social work, psychological, and nursing services, but the importance of medical—that is, psychiatric—care is evident.

The remaining 25 percent included personality disorders, sociopathic and dyssocial behaviors, alcoholism, a few cases of mental retardation, and two diagnosed as no mental illness. It seems to me that these are types of human difficulty with which psychiatry has not been notably successful, and it may well be that other mental health disciplines have more to offer. Reverting for a moment to the students at our School of Public Health, one gets the impression that when they are speaking of mental health problems, they are thinking mainly of this 25 percent, or are perhaps applying ideas that might be appropriate to some of this 25 percent to all 100 percent.

Table 1—2 shows the referral sources for the adult first admissions to the clinic. In 1952, 92 percent of referrals came from the medical system in the society of the geographic area, while 6 percent from informal community sources (that is, family, friends, and self). Fifteen years later, medical system referrals were still predominant, although they had dropped to 67 percent. The major percentage of increase was in referral from the community sources. Referrals from the social service systems were low at both points, in spite of a great increase in these services. It would seem, therefore, that referrals as well as syndrome types have something to say about the role of medicine in the care of the mentally ill as well as its relationships to other mental health disciplines.

One additional finding may be mentioned without resort to tables.

Table 1—2. Referral Sources of New Admission Adult Patients Seen in 1952 and 1967

Referral Source	1952		1967	
	No.	%	No.	%
Self, family, friend	(5)	6	(13)	20
Medical System: M.D., nurse, hospital	(74)	91	(42)	67
Social Systems: Church, court, welfare, other	(2)	3	(8)	13
Total	(81)	100	(63)	100

I shift attention now from patients attending the clinic to people in a probability sample of the population who were given mental illness ratings in 1952. A followup study in 1967 was able to show a relationship between death by 1967 and a mental illness rating in 1952 (Murphy, 1977). Those with serious mental illness ratings, particularly psychoses, had a considerably higher mortality rate than those who had been judged well.

This has some relevance to the issues of deinstitutionalization. Many studies have shown that patients in mental hospitals have a higher mortality rate than that which occurs in the population generally. Our findings suggest that mentally ill persons in the community also have a high rate. The point deserves investigation by other workers because if it is generally true it calls into question some of the claims made for deinstitutionalization.

These examples may perhaps serve to illustrate what Benjamin Franklin called "useful knowledge" as applied to community psychiatry. They also illustrate that only a beginning has been made in securing longitudinal information that is objective, systematic, reliable, and quantitative.

The Need to Study Communities

So far, I have spoken of the need for greater emphasis on the scientific study of mentally ill individuals in order to understand the effects of services. There is, however, another major topic of equal importance that can only be mentioned briefly in the space allotted. This is *the need to study communities*, sociologically and anthropologically, in order to understand how their patterning and functioning affect the success and failure of mental health service programs. There are many popular beliefs about the capabilities of communities that are based more on tradition and romantic hope than on what actually obtains today.

For example, in many towns both large and small a substantial portion of the population is transient. The resultant turnover every few years has serious implications for sustained participation in voluntary organizations, particularly since it is often those who can provide leadership, such as engineers, clergy, lawyers, and local managers for large companies, who are most apt to move. People who do not expect to be in a community for more than four or five years may give attention to short range projects, or to the schools, since these have immediate importance to their children, while long range programs tend to elicit less interest.

Another matter of significance is that communities are spread over a wide range of difference in terms of their degree of organizational cohesion, social integration, and morale. Many plans for the development of mental health programs have been launched without assessment as to whether the relevant communities have appropriate leadership and organizational capability. Techniques for these kinds of studies are in need of major development. Our experience suggests, unfortunately, that is is easy for mental health planners to have unrealistic expectations of communities.

Chapter 2

The Epidemiology
of Mental Illness

Psychiatric Epidemiology as a
Knowledge Base for Primary
Prevention in Community
Psychiatry and Community
Mental Health

Bruce P. Dohrenwend

Epidemiology is generally defined as the study of the occurrence (prevalence and incidence), distribution, and determinants of states of health in a population. Concern with populations distinguishes epidemiology from other medical studies that deal with individuals and their systems. Concern with states of health distinguishes epidemiological investigations from research focused on other characteristics of populations. Within the framework of these general distinctions (cf. Susser, 1968), psychiatric epidemiology consists of investigations of the kinds of phenomena that come under such headings as "mental health" and "mental disorders." It thus shares with the more policy and service oriented field of community mental health a focus on what Kessler and Albee (1975) have wryly described as "conditions which are not clearly defined, which vary in rate enormously as a function of community tolerance for deviance, which change frequencies with changing social conditions, and which may not even exist as identifiable individual defects" (p. 560).

In abstract, the relationship between psychiatric epidemiology and community mental health should be symbiotic. The main aim of

This work was supported by Research Grant MH 10328 and by Research Scientist Award K5–MH 14663 from the National Institute of Mental Health, U.S. Public Health Service.

The terms "community mental health" and "community psychiatry" will be used almost interchangeably in this paper. Where a particular author being referred to prefers one term or the other, that term will be used.

psychiatric epidemiology has been described by Cooper and Morgan (1973) as that of providing "a rational basis for preventive action" (p. 172). Complementary to this aim, Caplan has described the ultimate goal of community psychiatry as that of "lowering the rate of new cases of mental disorder in a population." (1964, p. 26). A basic assumption in community psychiatry and community mental health about how this goal is to be achieved involves "a view of mental disorder as rooted in the social system" (Smith and Hobbes, 1966, p. 9) and a belief that the pathogenic forces are mainly socioenvironmental (cf. Caplan and Grunebaum, 1967; Duhl, 1965; Glidewell, 1972; Cowen, 1973; Kessler and Albee, 1975). Critics have argued, however, that hard evidence for this assumption that socioenvironmental factors are important in the etiology of the so-called functional psychiatric disorders is lacking (e.g., Dunham, 1965; Wagonfeld, 1972).

Both their critics and those who have been at the forefront of the community mental health movement would agree on the inadequacy of the knowledge base. But adequacy and inadequacy are matters of degree. I am not at all sure what most workers in the field of community mental health believe that psychiatric epidemiology has shown, or failed to show, about relations between sociocultural and social psychological factors on the one hand, and mental disorders on the other. My purpose in this paper, therefore, will be to summarize my own assessment of the state of the evidence. In doing so, I will rely heavily on recent analyses of the epidemiological studies that Barbara Dohrenwend and I have done (B.P. Dohrenwend and B.S. Dohrenwend, 1974a; 1976) and also on some of our additional analyses of research that is perhaps less purely epidemiological (B.P. Dohrenwend and B.S. Dohrenwend, in press; B.P. Dohrenwend, 1975). The focus will be on studies mainly of adult subjects since there are others here, far better equipped than I, who will be reporting on research with children and adolescents. I will also attempt to trace some of the implications of this research for programs in community mental health. In doing so, I will concentrate on primary prevention since a whole section of papers by others at this symposium will be dealing with the evaluation of treatment.

STATE OF THE EVIDENCE

Much of the difficulty in determining what the facts are about relations between psychiatric disorders and various social and cultural factors, let alone how to interpret these facts, stems from two sources. The first is that most studies have defined cases of psychiatric disorder in terms of admission to psychiatric treatment. Although operationally the clearest definition of a "case," this is also the one with the most ambiguous implications for our problem. Since treatment rates vary with the availability of facilities and with public attitudes toward their use (cf. B.P. Dohrenwend and B.S. Dohrenwend, 1969, pp. 5–7), either of these conditions can account for correlations between social and cultural factors and rates of psychiatric disorder, measured by number of cases in treatment. For this reason, correlations involving only treated cases may be seriously misleading when the issues concern the significance of social and cultural factors in etiology (cf. Kramer, Rosen and Willis, 1973, especially 353–354 and p. 440; Gruenberg, 1974, especially, p. 454). The problem is far from solved, however, when we turn to research on "true" rates.

There has always been speculation about the true rates of psychiatric disorders in general populations. Some of this speculation has been put forth as official fact. It was possible to read in the *New York Times* (1975), for example, that:

> Mental illness is "America's primary health problem," affecting at least 10 percent of the population, according to the National Institute of Mental Health. Of the 20 million persons who suffer from some form of mental illness, one-seventh receive psychiatric care, the agency said . . . (p. 49B).

Since separate figures from NIMH suggest that clinical depression alone affects 19 to 20 million people a year in this country (Bunney, 1972; WNET, 1975) we may infer that the 10 percent figure for overall "mental illness" is indeed regarded as an underestimate.

I don't know where these figures come from, but they have clearly been produced under pressure. Before introducing them, the NIMH report on which the N.Y. Times release was based stated that "fully reliable statistics describing the incidence and prevalence of mental and emotional disorders do not exist" (Research Task Force of the National Institute of Mental Health, 1975, p. 3). And, as is stated flatly in the section of the report devoted to Biometry and Epidemiology, "Practical and reliable case-finding techniques do not exist" (p. 69). The fact of the matter is that once we decide not to rely on whether a person is in psychiatric treatment to define a "case," there is no clear consensus as to what should be included under such terms as "psychopathology," "psychiatric disorder," or "mental illness" or on how these phenomena should be measured. Herein lies the second major obstacle to determining what the facts are about; relations between sociocultural factors and psychiatric disorders.

Results from the "True" Prevalence Studies
of Psychiatric Disorders with No Known
Organic Basis

Despite these difficulties, about 60 different investigators or teams of investigators since the turn of the century have attempted to count not only treated cases but also untreated cases in over 80 studies (B.P. Dohrenwend and B.S. Dohrenwend, 1974a). These "true" prevalence studies have been conducted in communities all over the world—in North America, South America, Europe, Asia and Africa. With very few exceptions, the studies are cross-sectional in nature and the rates reported represent prevalence (the number of cases existing regardless of time of onset) during a period of a few months to a few years. Typically, the whole population in a specified geographical area is included in each of the investigations. Where studies have relied on sample estimates, the samples have usually been large. And when information has been provided on which "cases" were in treatment and which were not, the results have indicated that only small minorities were ever psychiatric patients (e.g., Srole et al., 1962; B.P. Dohrenwend, 1970).

The legacy from these epidemiological studies of true prevalence comes in two parts. The first, as might be anticipated from the discussion above, is a host of methodological problems centering on differences in how to conceptualize and measure "cases" of psychiatric disorder independently of treatment status. You can get some idea of the magnitude of the problem from the range in overall rates of functional psychiatric disorders reported in these studies. In some communities, rates of one percent and less were reported; in others, rates of 50 percent and more (B.P. Dohrenwend and B.S. Dohrenwend, 1974a, p. 423). Moreover, the differences are far more a function of contrasts in thoroughness of data collection procedures and, especially, contrasting conceptions about how to define a case than they are a function of substantive differences in the persons and places studied or the times at which the studies were conducted.

Thus, for example, considering only studies that used the more thorough data collection procedure of direct interviews with all subjects, we get the following differences in the medians of the overall rates for functional psychiatric disorders: 3.6 percent for the 6 such studies published before 1950 by contrast with about 18 percent for the 47 such studies published in 1950 or after. The tremendous increase is not a function of the increasing stresses and strains of the times in which we live. Rather, it is a function of the tremendous expansion of psychiatric nomenclatures on the basis of the experiences with psychiatric screening during World War II (cf. Raines, especially p. vi). Such expansion has led not only to an increase in the types of disorder included in diagnostic manuals, but also to a broadening of the definition of previously included types (cf. B.P. Dohrenwend and B.S. Dohrenwend, 1976).

These contrasts in concepts and methods render attempts to draw substantive conclusions from comparisons of absolute rates of various types of disorders reported by different investigators frustrating and uninformative (cf. B.P. Dohrenwend and B.S. Dohrenwend, 1974a, especially pp. 421–427). Despite these difficulties, there is a second part of the legacy from these studies that is all the more impressive because of the methodological differences. This second part of the legacy is a set of highly consistent *relationships* between various types of psychiatric disorders and such social factors as sex, social class, and urban by contrast with rural location. These relationships are all the more remarkable in that they hold across studies done at different times, in different parts of the world, and using different procedures for identifying cases. They provide the nearest things to the truth that we have from the epidemiological studies of "true" prevalence. Three sets of variables are involved in these relationships with psychiatric disorder: Sex, rural versus urban location, and social class. Let me summarize each in turn and describe the major issues of explanation that are posed.

Sex. The majority of the epidemiological studies of true prevalence have provided at least some data on psychiatric disorders according to sex. With *time* since the turn of the century specified as pre-World War II studies in which narrow definitions of psychiatric disorder tended to be used by contrast with post-World War II studies in which psychiatric definitions tended to be broader, and with *place* specified as rural and urban settings in selected North American and European communities by contrast with selected communities in the rest of the world, the firm facts that we have been able to extract (B.P. Dohrenwend and B.S. Dohrenwend, 1976) can be summarized as follows:

—There are no consistent sex differences in rates of functional psychoses in general (34 studies) or in rates of one of the two major subtypes, schizophrenia (26 studies) in particular; rates of the other, manic-depressive psychosis, are generally higher among women (18 out of 24 studies).

—Rates of neurosis are consistently higher for women regardless of time or place (28 out of 32 studies).

—By contrast, rates of personality disorder are consistently higher for men regardless of time or place (22 out of 26 studies).

The major issue here is posed by the relatively high female rates of neurosis and manic-depressive psychosis with their possible common denominator of depressive symptomatology (cf. Silverman, 1968; Klerman and Barrett, 1973), and the relatively high male rates of personality disorder with its possible common denominator or irresponsible and anti-social behavior (e.g., D.C. Leighton et al., especially p. 266 and p. 269; Robins, 1966, especially pp. 82–83; Mazer, 1974). The issue is: What is there in the endowments and experiences of men and women that push them in these different deviant directions? The problem in devising strategies to investigate this issue is the venerable and difficult one of how to isolate the influences of biological differences on the one hand, and differences in social role on the other. Progress waits on the development of such strategies.

Rural Versus Urban Settings. Given the differences in concepts and methods used in identifying cases in the true prevalence studies, comparisons of rate differences across studies done in rural and urban settings by different investigators is an exercise in futility. Fortunately, however, at least eight investigators have reported data for *both* a rural and an urban setting, with two reporting data for two settings each (B.P. Dohrenwend and B.S. Dohrenwend, 1974b). Here we have pairs of comparisons in which the same methodology was used to investigate the rural and urban subjects within each pair. Thus, although the between pair comparisons are not substantively meaningful, the within pair comparisons are, and once again we could search for trends.

In summary, we found that in one comparison, the total rate for all psychiatric disorders combined is higher in the rural setting; there is one tie; and in the remaining eight comparisons, the urban rate is higher than the rural rate. Although quite consistent, however, the differences are not large; the median difference for total rates is only 1.1 percent and the range is from an excess of 0.9 percent in a rural area to an excess of 13.9 percent in an urban area. The reason is that while some types of psychiatric disorder were found to be more prevalent in the urban setting, others were found more frequently in the rural setting. Thus:

—Total rates for all functional psychoses combined were found to be more prevalent in the rural settings (5 out of 7 studies), and this appears to be so for the manic-depressive subtype (3 out of 4 studies), though not for schizophrenia (higher in the urban area in 3 out of 5 studies).

—Rates of neurosis were higher in the urban settings (5 out of 6 studies).

—Rates of personality disorder were higher in the urban settings (5 out of 6 studies).

While some of these results are consistent with popular speculations about the pathological consequences of stressful urban environments, they are also consistent with plausible alternative interpretations. However harsh and threatening cities may be, they also provide concentrations of industry and commerce, wealth and power, and art and entertainment that make them magnets for rural people. Migrants seeking greater opportunity, challenge, or, perhaps, anonymity are drawn to cities in large numbers. The possibility cannot be overlooked, therefore, that such migrants bring with them the types of psychopathology that show higher rates in urban settings. Unfortunately, no studies exist that have taken pre-migration baseline measures of "true" prevalence, followed up by post-migration measures in the urban destination. In the absence of such studies, this is another issue that remains unresolved.

Social Class. In 1855, Edward Jarvis, a physician in the state of Massachusetts, submitted a report on probably the most complete and influential attempt to investigate the true prevalence of psychiatric disorders conducted in the nineteenth century (Jarvis, 1971). This was almost half a century before the Kraepelinian era in psychiatry and the only nosological distinction that he made was between "insanity" and "idiocy." His main finding was the "the pauper class furnishes, in ratio of its numbers, 64 times as many cases of insanity as the independent class" (1971, pp. 52–53). This basic finding of the highest overall rate in the lowest social class has remained remarkably persistent in the true prevalence studies conducted since the turn of the century (B.P. Dohrenwend and B.S. Dohrenwend, 1974a):

—The highest overall rates of psychiatric disorder have been found in the lowest social class in 28 out of the 33 studies that report data, according to indicators of social class such as occupation, education, and income.

—This relationship is strongest in the studies conducted in urban settings or mixed urban and rural settings (19 out of 20 studies).

—The relationship holds for the important subtypes of schizophrenia (5 out of 7 studies) and personality disorder (11 out of 14 studies).

Jarvis thought he knew why the rates of insanity were highest in the lowest social class. He wrote in 1855:

Men of unbalanced mind and uncertain judgment do not see the true nature and relation of things, and they manifest this in mismanagement of their common affairs. They do not adapt the means which they possess or use to the ends which they desire to produce. Hence they are unsuccessful in life; their plans of obtaining subsistence for themselves or their families, or of accumulating property, often fail; and they are consequently poor, and often paupers . . . the cause of . . . their mental derangement lies behind, and is anterior to, their outward poverty (1971, pp. 55–56).

In this interpretation Jarvis provides an early example of what has come to be known as social selection explanations of relationships between social position and psychiatric disorder. It is the type of explanation involved in our earlier consideration of the possibility that rural migrants to cities may bring pathology with them rather than developing it in response to the stress of urban living.

The explanation of Jarvis is in sharp contrast with one that Faris and Dunham (1939) favored for their not dissimilar finding of disproportionately high rates of mental hospital first admissions, from the central slum sections of Chicago in the 1930s. Faris and Dunham wrote:

> In these most disorganized sections of the city and, for that matter, of our whole civilization, many persons are unable to achieve a satisfactory conventional organization of their world. The result may be lack of any organization at all, resulting in a confused, frustrated, and chaotic personality . . . (1939, p. 159).

Unfortunately, Faris and Dunham's views, like the contrasting views of Jarvis, were reflections more of the differing Zeitgeists, than a clear choice on the basis of the evidence between the opposing social stress and social selection explanations.

The class findings from the "true" prevalence studies summarized above, then, have served to raise and reraise the social stress–social selection issue—sometimes with more and sometimes with less sophistication. No research to date has resolved this issue in the sense of assessing the relative importance of the two processes (stress and selection) and the nature of their interaction in relations between social class and various types of psychiatric disorder (B.P. Dohrenwend, 1975).

It is possible to conceive, in the abstract, of straightforward approaches such as multigeneration prospective designs or experiments with humans that could resolve the issue. Such research has simply not been undertaken on practical and ethical grounds—although some recent and ongoing research involving shorter term followups of general population samples between five and twenty years after baseline data were collected, promises to yield important information on incidence (the number of new cases that occur within a given interval of time), that should help us to clarify the direction of the relationships between social class and various types of psychopathology (e.g., Hagnell, 1966; Gersten, et al., 1974; Beiser, 1971; and Srole, 1975).

Perhaps an example from another field will illustrate both the simplicity of a resolution in abstract and the difficulty in carrying it out in the real world of social and psychiatric research. The example has been provided by Thoday and Gibson (1970) who have conducted a fascinating model experiment showing not only how the stress-selection issue, but also how the larger environment-heredity issue that it implies, can be tested. Their subjects were nine generations of flies; the characteristic to be explained was the number of bristles that the flies would develop; and the environmental variable was temperature. The procedures included the use of a "transplant" or cross-over design and provision for an assessment of the effects of assortative mating. The result is an extraordinarily elegant experiment leading to clear-cut findings—insofar as bristles on flies are concerned. The important point, of course, is that the choice of flies, as subjects, enabled the investigators to solve all or most of the design problems, including that of history—the very problems that have constituted insurmountable practical and ethical difficulties when the subjects are humans and the effect in which we are interested consists of psychopathology.

It is my belief, therefore, that advances on this important issue are much more likely to come from indirect approaches that permit deductions on the basis of carefully thought out and investigated quasi-experiments of nature. Examples on the genetic side of the nature-nurture issue have been provided in the twin and adoption strategies so successfully employed in the study of schizophrenia (cf. Gottesman and Shields, 1972; Heston, 1966; Rosenthal and Kety, 1968). We have set forth the ingredients of what we hope is a promising quasi-experimental strategy based on socioenvironmental contrasts elsewhere (B.P. Dohrenwend, 1966; B.P. Dohrenwend and B.S. Dohrenwend, 1969; 1974b) and have reported intriguing findings from our own research and that of others that bear on the strategy (B.P. Dohrenwend, 1975). It is however, a long way from being fully implemented, and the basic issue of the relative importance of social stress and social selection in the class differences remains unresolved.

Physical Illness and Psychiatric Disorder

An increasing number of researchers have been investigating relations between episodes of physical illness and episodes of emotional disturbance (e.g., Hinkle and Wolff, 1957; Shepherd, Cooper, Brown and Kalton, 1966; Eastwood, 1975). For the most part, these investigations are not epidemiological studies of communities; rather, they are studies of patient populations in which the investigators often use case-control designs. They include, however, data from a wide variety of patients, ranging from those chosen on the basis of the presence of a particular type of physical illness or psychiatric disorder to the families comprising the patients of various general practitioners in Great Britain.

The findings from these diverse studies are remarkably consistent; there is a strong positive association between physical illness and psychiatric disorder (cf. Lipowski, 1975). On the basis of a detailed review of the literature Lipowski (1975) has concluded:

> Despite the high frequency and practical importance of this associa-
> tion . . . the whole area of psychopathology related to physical illness has
> been relatively neglected by American psychiatrists. We know little about
> the incidence and prevalence of psychiatric disorders caused by organic
> disease in general, and by the various classes of somatic disorder in particu-
> lar. . . . The mechanisms, processes and significant variables intervening
> between a given physical disorder or injury on the one hand and the devel-
> opment of psychological dysfunction on the other . . . are still inadequately
> worked out (p. 105).

Studies of Extreme Situations

The most persuasive evidence that environmentally induced stress is important in the causation of a wide variety of signs and symptoms of psychiatric disorder in substantial portions of the general population, is indirect. The reason is that this compelling evidence comes, not from the epidemiological studies of such populations under ordinary conditions, but rather from studies of individuals and groups under the extraordinary conditions imposed by natural and man-made disasters, especially the disaster of war.

On the basis of several reviews and analyses of the literature on extreme situations (B.P. Dohrenwend and B.S. Dohrenwend, 1969; in press), we have concluded, as others have done, that some circumstances will produce a wide variety of psychiatric signs and symptoms in all or most previously normal persons—in fact, even in persons selected for their high ability to cope with stressful situations.

For example, on the basis of a study of 2,630 soldiers who had broken down during combat in the Normandy campaign during World War II, Swank (1949) estimated that the onset of combat exhaustion occurred in previously normal soldiers when about 65 percent of their companions had been killed, wounded or had otherwise become casualties (p. 501). Nor are the symptoms caused by such situations of extreme stress limited to those included under the heading of traumatic war neurosis, combat fatigue, and combat exhaustion. There is evidence that psychotic symptoms can appear in the form of what have been called "three-day" psychoses (Kolb, 1973, p. 438). It is possible, in fact, that such extreme circumstances can play a major role in inducing outright psychotic disorder since, as Paster (1948) found, there is far less evidence of individual predisposing factors in combat soldiers who became psychotic, than among soldiers who developed psychotic disorders in less stressful circumstances. It would seem that a large portion of the signs and symptoms observed in psychiatric patients in civilian settings have also been observed in the form of reactions to combat (cf. Kolb, 1973, pp. 436—438).

Stressful Life Events

Natural and man-made disasters, fortunately, are rare occurrences, whose devastating effects are limited to relatively small populations of exposed persons. Most people live their lives without experiencing any of these extraordinary events. Yet, we have learned from the epidemiological studies of true prevalence that psychiatric symptoms are far from rare occurrences in peacetime populations relatively secure from war, flood, famine and other disasters. Especially in the studies conducted in 1950 or later and using broad definitions of what constitutes a case, substantial portions of the population—sometimes 50 percent and more—are judged to be suffering from psychiatric disorders (B.P. Dohrenwend and B.S. Dohrenwend, 1974a).

If stressful situations play an important etiological role in such psychopathology, the events involved must be more ordinary, more frequent experiences in the lives of most people. It is for this reason that it seems important to turn our attention to things that happen to most people at one time or another—things such as marriage, birth of a first child, physical illness, the death of a loved one. These are not extraordinary events in the sense of being of rare occurrence in most populations. But they are extraordinary occurrences in the lives of the individuals who experience them.

Most of these life events, taken singly, are far less extreme than natural or man-made disasters. One reason is that a disaster is likely to entail as sequalae a number of events all at the same time or closely spaced—injury, loss of home and other possessions, death of a loved one. It seems reasonable to assume that life events must show a cumulative pattern, a clustering in the lives of some people in more ordinary times if they are to have a similarly stressful impact and similarly severe consequences. Certainly, this is the implicit or explicit assumption on which most life events research with general populations has been based (cf. B.S. Dohrenwend and B.P. Dohrenwend, 1974a).

To date, however, the results of research on the influence of these more ordinary life events on various types of psychiatric conditions are far more equivocal than the results of research on the effects of natural and manmade disasters (cf. B.P. Dohrenwend and B.S. Dohrenwend, in press). Nevertheless, the results to date have yielded a fascinating set of correlations that, while often controversial as to interpretation, virtually demand further research (cf. B.S. Dohrenwend and B.P. Dohrenwend, 1974a). Moreover, the methodological issues posed by this research are becoming clearer, and major advances can be expected in the near future (cf. Brown, 1974; B.S. Dohrenwend and B.P. Dohrenwend, 1974b).

If environmentally induced stress is indeed an important factor in the etiology of various types of functional psychiatric disorder in general populations, then life events are strategic phenomena on which to focus as possible major sources of such stress. It is possible to envision, in fact, powerful research strategies developing in the form of convergences between quasi-experimental designs focused on explaining relations between gross social factors such as class and psychiatric disorders, and life events research that will place psychopathology in more specific situational contexts (cf. B.P. Dohrenwend, 1975).

PRIMARY PREVENTION

It is much easier for a researcher reviewing a field of investigation to talk about the implications for further research than about the implications for utilization or action. I see that this is, indeed, what I have done up to now. There are, however, some implications for primary prevention that I would like to consider. One of them involves the location of targets for action that seem compelling in terms of the sheer magnitude of the social problems involved. Some of the relationships with, for example, social class, are strong and consistent enough to tempt one to advocate a "miasma" removal approach to primary prevention. The argument would be that concentrations of psychopathology could be eliminated by the removal of poverty and slums (see Bloom, 1965; Kessler and Albee, 1975, p. 577). In Bloom's (1965) account, miasma theory dates from the writings of Hippocrates and precedes germ theories of the etiology of infectious diseases:

> It held that soil polluted with waste products of any kind gave off a "miasma" into the air, which caused many major infectious diseases of the day. This theory . . . suggested that these "poisonous substances" rose up from the earth and were spread through the winds (p. 334).

Bloom argues that, while miasma theory has been discredited, so far as etiology is concerned, it nevertheless led to tremendously effective preventive actions by sanitarians and engineers. He suggests that, given our very incomplete knowledge of the causes of the functional psychiatric disorders, such a theory might be most appropriate as a basis for preventive efforts in community mental health.

Durkheim's (1951) notion of "anomie" and more recent concepts such as Faris and Dunham's (1939) "social disorganization" and the "social disintegration" theory of A.H. Leighton (1959) seem to me to be twentieth century counterparts in the behavioral sciences to the nineteenth century miasma theory of the sanitarians. There is some evidence from the research of Leighton and his colleagues in Stirling County that social change of a sufficient magnitude to transform a community from a disorganized and poverty stricken one to a relatively well off and stable one will indeed alter its rate of psychiatric disorder (A.H. Leighton, 1965). Note, however, that the example from Stirling County is a rare one. It centered on a very small rural neighborhood that had been closely observed by the research team over a period of more than ten years. This research setting is hardly typical of the sociocultural miasmas that develop in our modern, urban centers; nor is the committment to long term research and the good fortune to have a major social and economic change occur during it, typical of our research enterprises in psychiatric epidemiology.

As to the role of the community mental health professions with regard to bringing about planned changes of such magnitude, they simply have neither the power nor the right. As Kessler and Albee (1975, p. 577) point out, the preventive efforts of the sanitarians and engineers guided by the miasma theory involved relatively little threat to the social order. This, of course, would not be the case for community mental health professionals interested in preventive efforts modeled on a behavioral science counterpart to miasma theory. It seems to me, therefore, that the behavioral science analogies to miasma theory are more suitable as ideological bases for political action, even revolution, than for preventive efforts by mental health professionals (cf. Kessler and Albee, 1975, pp. 577–578).

The fact remains, however, that rarely if ever will a disease or disorder be eradicated from a population by efforts at treating or rehabilitating people who have become afflicted. Moreover, political revolutions have had a tendency to replace the miasmas they remove with others that are no less unattractive. Fortunately, however, research results already available suggest a more specific target, one centered more on the individual and his or her concerns than on the larger social systems in which the individual participates. This is the research on stressful life events.

To the extent to which further research shows that an appreciable portion of the signs and symptoms observed in general populations are reactions to stressful life events, including, and perhaps especially, physical illness and injury, additional and highly intriguing possibilities for primary prevention will occur. The sequence of causation for such disorder would have much in common with that observed in combat reactions, with similar possibilities for locating clues to the effective prevention of severe reactions and chronic course (see, for example, Glass, 1969 by contrast with Caplan and Grunebaum, 1967).

It would be foolish, however, to overestimate the ease of extrapolating from the combat situation in wartime to the stressful events of everyday life. As Grinker and Spiegel (1963) wrote on the basis of their research during World War II:

> ... war is a natural experiment—a laboratory which manufactures psychological dysfunction at an appalling rate. There is no other situation which guarantees such easily observed failures of adaptive function in such large numbers under such standardized conditions. ... The relation between endopsychic, predispositional factors and the external, social factors is usually easy to assess. The vagueness of the ordinary human predicament which makes the environmental variables so difficult to estimate in most circumstances is replaced by the dramatic contingencies of the combat situation (1963, pp. vii–viii).

It is, however, the "vagueness of the ordinary human predicament" that we must attempt to clarify in research on life events in general populations.

Many of the life events with which we are concerned, events such as divorce or loss of a job, can occur as concomitants or consequences of the individual's psychiatric condition. Even results from prospective studies, where the temporal sequence between such events and symptomatology are better established, can be problematic with regard to causal inference because so many of the psychiatric disorders are of insidious onset. In the combat situation, the fatefulness of the events experienced, the extent to which their occurrence is objectively within or outside the control of the individual soldier, is usually self-evident. This is sometimes so for more usual life events such as death of a loved one; but often, as in the examples above of divorce and loss of a job, this is not the case. The central problem for further research on life events, therefore, is how to measure their stressfulness independent of the psychiatric condition of the subjects.

It is failure to come to terms with this problem that is responsible for much of the ambiguity in the results of research on relations between life events and psychopathology (cf. Langner, 1963; Brown, 1974; B.P. Dohrenwend, 1974; B.S. Dohrenwend and B.P. Dohrenwend, 1974b; B.P. Dohrenwend and B.S. Dohrenwend, in press).

IN CONCLUSION

If the past is any guide to the future, predictions about what we will know "x" years from now about the causes of the functional psychiatric disorders are hazardous. Will there be a vaiable knowledge base for preventive action from the standpoint of a socioenvironmental orientation to etiology in the forseeable future? I don't know. If there is, I think that it will emerge from the study of stressful life events within a wider framework of epidemiological investigation.

The Epidemiology of Mental Disorder in Children: Implications for Community Psychiatry

Thomas S. Langner
Joanne C. Gersten
Jeanne G. Eisenberg

Though there are children's mental disorders which are heavily organic or genetic in origin, I will not cover them here. Not only is this not my area of expertise, but the disorders are relatively rare when compared with those suspected of being primarily psychosocial in origin. The great improvement in children with mild mental retardation, spontaneously or after exposure to early stimulation or cognitive training programs, suggests that with the exception of extreme cases, there is a large social component even in disorders which are considered heavily genetic. (Stein & Susser, 1970, 1971).

Childhood psychoses are also very rare, since they are estimated to occur in about six out of 10,000 cases—six hundredths of 1 percent. In contrast, apprehended antisocial behavior measured in a longitudinal survey, which my colleagues and I have conducted in New York City, was found in 20 percent of all boys in the general population (a rate of period prevalence). This is 333 times the average prevalence

This investigation was supported by U.S. Public Health Service Project Grants MH 11545 and MH 18260 of the National Institute of Mental Health, Center for Epidemiologic Studies, by the U.S. Department of Health, Education, and Welfare, Social and Rehabilitation Service, Cooperative Research and Demonstration Grants Branch, grant SRS–CRD–348 (SRS–56006), and by the Office of Child Development, grants OCD–CB–348 and OCD–CB–480.

Support for the principal investigator was given by Career Scientist Awards I–338 and I–640 of the Health Research Council of the City of New York. The principal investigator is currently supported through Research Scientist Award K5–MH–20868 of the National Institute of Mental Health.

The authors would like to express their gratitude to Elizabeth D. McCarthy, M.A., who has helped in all phases of the research project. Dr. Ora Simcha-Fagan, who is analyzing project data on drug abuse and violence, supplied appropriate data for this paper. Drs. Edward L. Greene, Joseph H. Herson, and Jean D. Jameson contributed to the work by making psychiatric evaluations of the children. Ms. Nathalia Lange served as field director of the project. Drs. Jacob and Patricia Cohen contributed valuable statistical advice in an earlier phase of the project.

rate of psychoses. In terms of both frequency and seriousness for the child and the community, it deserves primary consideration.

From the standpoint of theory and of their own etiology, it is important to study childhood psychoses, but they do not necessarily predict adult psychoses (Achenbach, 1974). Yolles and Kramer (1969) found that the rates of adult psychosis varied between 380 and 2,350 per 10,000 or from 3.8 to 23.5 percent; the latter reported in rural Sweden. Thus the rates for adult psychosis vary up to about 400 times as great as those of children. Such types as Kanner's autistic children (Kanner, 1943) are so rare that it is difficult to find a large series of cases. Kanner (1971), Eisenberg (1956), and others (Kanner, Rodrigues, and Ashenden, 1971) found only 11 of 96 diagnosed autistic children to be functioning at all adequately in adult life. These rare conditions are serious, and deserve twin and high risk studies such as those on schizophrenia.

The etiology of these conditions seems to be highly specific, however. For example, pregnancy and birth complications correlate with poor infant developmental scores *only* in children of schizophrenics, not in children of nonschizophrenics, leaving us with the impression that there is an interaction effect of birth complications with some genetic vulnerability (Mednick and Schulzinger, 1972). Out of a total of 524 children of schizophrenic parents in three high risk studies, none was diagnosed as a childhood schizophrenic. Some 10 to 20 percent may be expected to be schizophrenic as adults, however (Achenbach, 1974).

While children's disorders need prevention and intervention in their own right, their predictivity for adult dysfunction is an important consideration. According to Robins (1966), the prediction of adult antisocial behavior from children's antisocial behavior is relatively accurate. A group of 524 adults who had been in a psychiatric clinic as children, were matched with controls. Patients exceeded controls in all measures of adult antisocial behavior. One fourth of the children referred for antisocial reasons were later diagnosed as having adult sociopathic personality. No child was later diagnosed as a sociopath who did not show such behavior earlier. The 25 percent consistency rate compares favorably with the rates of schizophrenia in children of schizophrenic parents.

It is generally believed that social and psychological forces are much more important in criminality than are genetic forces. Robins found that if the child's father was a sociopath, the risk of the child's being antisocial was greatly increased. This was also true if the father had died or abandoned the family either before the child's birth or very early in life. This might seem to favor the genetic hypothesis, and challenge the sociogenic hypothesis that the father always acts as the sociopathic model for the child.

We have been able to test the idea that the mother of the anti-social child may have covert antisocial tendencies herself, which were involved in her initial selection of an antisocial mate who acted out her impulses, and which would influence her child rearing in that area. A series of scales measuring mothers antisocial attitudes show that her violent feelings do help to predict violence in her children. (There were several dimensions of mother's attitudes constructed which were felt to be potentially related to violent child behavior. These were correlated with the presence or absence of all siblings in the family on criminal records as follows: Nontraditionalism, Pearson r = .19; Fatalism-Suspiciousness, r = .18; Puritan Ethic, r = .16).

It is also misleading to study uncommon child disorders in an attempt to unravel the etiology of the more common disorders. For example; we have found a strong set of predictors for heroin abuse (Multiple R = .77; % variance = .60) in our study, while there seems to be a less well defined set of predictors for the more widespread phenomenon of marijuana use (R = .55; % variance = .30). The rate of heroin use was 7 percent, while that of marijuana use was 54 percent.

THE DEPENDENT VARIABLES: DEFINING DISORDER

Further progress in uncovering the causes of behavioral disorder in children, even more than in adults, is hampered by the lack of any reliable classification system. Despite great effort, the ability of clinicians to agree to judgments on known patients, using the common diagnostic categories, has on average been quite low. Some typical agreement coefficients are, for depression, around .30 (Zubin, Salzinger, et al., 1975), for schizophrenia and affective psychoses, .59 (Fleiss, Spitzer, Endicott and Cohen, 1972). For specific APA nomenclature categories, agreement ranged from .06 to .49, averaging .30 (Zubin et al., 1975). There is a parallel to Kessler & Albee's question "If we cannot define mental illness reliably, how can we prevent it?" Just as true is the question, "If we cannot define mental health, how can we foster or promote it?"

There are two different approaches to classification (Lorr, 1961); a class model and a quantitative model. The older adult and child diagnostic systems are typical of class models, since the categories are considered to be mutually exclusive and to have different etiologies and life courses. Thus one cannot be considered both psychotic and neurotic simultaneously. Most of the symptoms must be evident before the disorder can be present. The quantitative model, on the other hand, considers the disorder to be not merely present or absent, but graded upon a continuum of intensity, dependent upon the number of symptoms of that particular dimension found present.

I think our research, not unlike some other more recent research, has bridged this apparently insoluble gap between class and continuous models, by use of readily available methodology. It seems reasonable that the end product of classification for most practical purposes should be an individual, not a continuum. The clinician, as opposed to the pure researcher, wants some*body*, not something, he can refer for treatment, or send home.

Since I will be giving many examples of findings and problems from our research, a very brief description is necessary here. The Family Research Project, including its planning, has been in progress for ten years. Presently a team composed of three sociologists, one psychologist, and one social worker, with other supporting personnel, remain on the staff, which originally included three psychiatrists who evaluated the children by direct examination and by means of summarized reports from the mothers. Two samples were studies; the first was a representative sample of 1034 children aged 6 to 18 selected randomly from a cross-section of Manhattan (New York City) households between Houston and 125th Streets.

A stratified systematic cluster sampling plan resulted in a sample that was 56 percent white, 14 percent black, 29 percent Spanish-speaking, and 1 percent other. The second sample consisted of 1000 children aged 6 to 18 who were members of households receiving Aid to Dependent Children. The households were randomly selected within ethnic groups from welfare rolls in the same geographic area as the cross-section sample. About equal thirds of black, white and Spanish-speaking households were chosen, so that adequate numbers of each ethnic group would be available for comparisons. Each age group comprised nearly one-thirteenth of each of the samples, and males and females were fairly evenly distributed across the thirteen age groups.

Mothers were interviewed in the selected households for two to three hours using a structured questionnaire about the chosen child and the family. The survey completion rate was 85 percent. Children were rated on ten 5-point scales of impairment by at least two of the psychiatrists, using a computer summary of the 654 items of information on the child's behavior given by the mother, with a reliability for the average of two raters of .84 for the most global rating. Direct psychiatric examinations were given to 271 cross-section and 86 welfare children, and ratings made on the same dimensions. The mean correlations between the ratings made on mother's report, and ratings made on direct examination, were .48 by Pearson product moment and .33 by intraclass correlation.

The method discussed below shows how one can convert dimensions of behavior back into people, or shift from the quantitative back to the class model, or to quasi-diagnostic categories, when necessary. This also suggests that resistance to dimensional or quantitative research on the grounds that it cannot be understood by those who give services to adults or children because it uses dimensions, not people, is groundless at this date.

A disorder is, of course, not made up of one continuum, but several. It was possible to reduce a large pool of 654 behavior items by eliminating symptoms which were not correlated strongly with any underlying dimension, those which were extremely rare, and those which were exclusively contingent upon age, sex, or other demographic categories.

Of the 654 items, about 200 were collapsed into a series of composite scores (e.g., number of fears, number of illnesses). From the reduced pool of 287 items, a sample of items representing symptoms from various organ systems, behavior areas, behavior settings, and relationships to specific family figures was chosen from a group of symptoms judged more serious than others. These were about half of the reduced pool. They were factored by using principal components with varimax rotation to create marker variables, and placed in a second matrix with the less serious half.

In a series of similar procedures, 221 items were finally formed into 18 relatively independent dimensions of child behavior, with relatively high reliability or internal consistency. These factored dimensions, listed in order of decreased reliability, were Conflict with Parents, Dependence, Fighting, Regressive Anxiety, Mentation Problems, Competition, Delinquency, Self-Destructive Tendencies, Undemandingness, Conflict with Siblings, Isolation, Repetitive Motor Behavior, Non-Complusive, Sex Curiosity, Training Difficulties, Weak Group Membership, Delusions-Hallucinations, and Late Development. Reliability ranged from .94 to .69 (see Table 2–1).

We standardized these dimensions, and then subjected them to Hierarchical Cluster Analysis (McKeon, 1967). This is a procedure which in a sense tells the computer to take the first child's profile over these 18 dimensions and search until it finds a mate which is closest to this child. Then the two children form a group which seeks a third child, until certain internal limits are exceeded, whereupon a

Table 2-1.   The Eighteen Child Behavior Factors, with Representative Items and Their Factor Loadings and the Reliability Coefficient of the Factor

Factor	Content	Correlation with Factor Score	Reliability Coefficient
1 Sex Curiosity (*N = 7)	Masturbates often Likes to see parents undressed	.65 .59	.76
2 Self-Destructive Tendencies (N = 6)	Talks about killing himself now Talked about death recently	.72 .67	.84
3 Mentation Problems (N = 21)	Mixes up words and has Trouble remembering things	.54 .50	.87
4 Conflict with Parents (N = 38)	Often blows up easily with Mother and Father	.62 .57	.94
5 Dependence-Unassertiveness (N = 9)	Never acts independently of Mother and Father	.76 .74	.92
6 Regressive Anxiety (N = 24)	Has many fears Often wakes up in a panic	− .51 .49	.88
7 Group Membership Weak (N = 6)	Is not a member of an organized group nor an officer	.59 .54	.73
8 Non-Compulsive (N = 15)	Never checks on things several times nor is concerned with being on time	− .55 − .51	.77
9 Training Difficulties (N = 7)	Late bladder control and Late bowel control	.60 .59	.75
10 Undemandingness (N = 6)	Never asks mother to be taken places or to spend time with him	.82 .79	.84

11	Repetitive Motor Behavior (N = 7)	Often whirls, spins and bangs his head	.65 .61	.78
12	Fighting (N = 21)	Teases other children and does not get along with other children at school	.57 .56	.90
13	Delusions-Hallucinations (N = 7)	Hears peculiar sounds or voices in head / Sees, hears, smells things others do not	.63 .56	.72
14	Competition with Others (N = 4)	Often competes with Father and Mother	.76 .74	.87
15	Delinquency (N = 19)	Smokes and Plays hookey	.56 .55	.86
16	Conflict with Siblings (N = 10)	Blows up easily with sibs and often expresses anger toward them	.68 .66	.83
17	Late Development (N = 6)	Began to walk late and hardly moved about at all as a baby	-.56 -.55	.69
18	Isolation (N = 9)	Often plays alone and doesn't keep a friend a year or more	.56 .55	.79

*N is the number of items in the factor.

new group is formed and goes recruiting. The model for this system is based upon the sum of each child's squared distances from the initial average profiles in his own three-year age group.

This system has allowed us to retain the dimensions of behavior which are so necessary to basic research, but it also allows us to regroup these dimensions once again into actual people. The examination of peaks and valleys of the average profiles which are 1/2 to 1 standard deviation from the mean, allows us to give names to the children who fall into those types. For example, children who showed more conflict with parents and siblings, more fighting, more delinquency, more independence, and less compulsivity than their age peers were labeled "Aggressive." They constituted 12 percent of the random sample.

The profile or H types can be pretty well identified by their names. Their prevalence in the random sample is also given, rounded off to the nearest whole percent. They are: Sociable 16%, Competitive-Independent 12%, Dependent 34%, Moderate Backward Isolate 16%, Aggressive 12%, Severe Backward Isolate 4%, Organic 1%, Other 2%. This material is shown in Table 2−2.

Getting back to whole children, rather than parts, we can check our classification system against external criteria, never forgetting that these are open to many biases and distortions. As an example, let's take the children identified as Aggressive by their profiles. Many of these children and adolescents are known to the police, courts, and other social agencies. We are now searching these records, including school records, which allows us to calibrate these dimensions and profiles with what we used to consider "hard data." It is now common knowledge that only a small portion of delinquents and criminals are apprehended. The ratio of unreported crime to reported crime (survey vs. police data) ranges from 5.1:1 to 1.4:1 for thirteen large U.S. cities (Burnham, 1974). Moreover, a severe race and class bias exists among the apprehended.

Referral and treatment for behavior problems is another indicator by which we can attempt to interpret, if not to calibrate, our proportions of Aggressive children. What proportion of the Aggressives are arrested, convicted, treated, injured, abused? These types of children can be counted, new samples of children can be classified into these types with very little error, and parental reports (or the child's own reports in the case of older children) can be used alternatively. Ideally these types should be based upon detailed observations of children in different behavioral settings over a long period of time. It would make me feel very secure to see a congruence between self or parent reports, case records, and the report of observers. Given the current state of research funding, I don't think we can expect detailed observations on a thousand or two thousand children, and a factoring and profiling of their behavior, for some time to come.

Our current data indicate good agreement between the mean levels of behavior reported by mothers and children. Only children 14 years or older reported on their own behavior. *T*-tests were made for the factor means on sixteen child behavior dimensions. There was no mean difference between children and mothers on seven factors, including Conflict with Parents, Dependence, and Conflict with Siblings. Children had higher scores on eight other factors, including Anxiety, Delinquency, and Fighting. Lapouse and Monk (1958) found greater proportions of children than mothers reporting symptoms concerned with mood and affect, which is reflected in our higher child reports of Anxiety.

Presumably not all moods, or ideation, are communicated to the parents. Children were also expected to report, and did report, more antisocial behavior outside the home, since this was a setting which the mother could not usually observe. However, the correlation between the two reporters was only .40 or greater for six of the sixteen factors, the best agreement being .79 for Delinquency, which was unexpected.

There are thus fairly low levels of agreement between the rank ordering of the children as reported by themselves and their mothers. Agreement varies by ethnic background; Spanish-speaking mothers and children agreed more than whites, who in turn agreed more than blacks. Spanish respondents agreed with a correlation of .40 or better on eight dimensions, blacks on only four. Using the same criterion, mothers with eight years or less of education agreed with their children on eight dimensions, those with high school education (9 to 12 years) agreed on seven, and college level or better agreed on only six.

Ethnic differences, as in all our data, seem stronger than socioeconomic ones, even in other cases in which there is partialling of effects. Agreement checks with school, police, court, and social agency data are now in progress. In different behavior settings we expect real differences in child behavior. If behaviors were limited to one setting, the home, there might be higher correlations. One thing is certain—mothers *did* underreport by comparison with their older children, so our estimates of psychopathology are conservative.

Table 2-2.   Child H Types (Profiles): Child Factors with Z Scores ≥ .50 Within Each Child Type and Percentage of Children with Total Impairment Rating of 4+.

Child Types	Type Exhibits Less Of	Type Exhibits More Of	% Rated 4 & 5	% of Sample
Sociable	Weak group membership[a]	—	1.7	16.2
Competitive-Independence	Dependence Training difficulties	Competitiveness	1.6	11.5
Dependent	Regressive anxiety Conflict with parents	—	1.4	34.3
Moderate Backward—Isolate	—	Late development Isolation	15.4	15.7
Aggressive	Dependence	Conflict with parents Sex curiosity Fighting Conflict with siblings	22.4	12.0
Severe Backward Isolate	—	Repetitive Motor Behavior[a] Isolation[a] Late development Conflict with parents Mentation problems Regressive anxiety Delinquency Training difficulties Fighting	40.5	3.6
Delusional	Noncompulsive	Delusions-Hallucinations[a] Regressive anxiety Delinquency Isolation	53.3	1.5

Self and Other Destructive	—	Self-destructive tendencies[a] Fighting[a] Conflict with parents[a] Regressive anxiety[a] Delinquency[a] Mentation problems[a] Isolation Conflict with siblings Late development Sex curiosity	58.5	2.8
Organic	Dependence	Mentation problems[a] Delusions-Hallucinations[a] Regressive anxiety[a] Isolation[a] Fighting[a] Late development[a] Repetitive motor behavior[a] Conflict with parents[a] Conflict with siblings[a] Training difficulties Competitiveness Delinquency	57.1	0.7
Other	Noncompulsive	Delinquency[a] Fighting[a] Delusions-Hallucinations[a] Conflict with parents[a] Training difficulties[a] Mentation problems[a] Conflict with siblings[a] Regressive anxiety Isolation Dependence	61.1	1.7

100% = 1,034

[a] = 1 or more standard deviation units.

THE INDEPENDENT VARIABLES

Predictors of Children's Disorder, and Possible Intervention Points

The number of studies of factors that might cause different types of behavioral, psychiatric, or developmental disorders in children is truly astronomical. While there are some outstanding and deservedly first magnitude studies in this "Milky Way" of publication, the different methods and sources, and the different frameworks and classification systems of the investigators, make firm statements about our state of knowledge difficult, though not impossible. Most problematic of all is the fact that few studies of any size have been conducted on random samples of children, have used multidimensional dependent and independent variables, and have ranked predictors by predictive power.

The implications for prevention and for community psychiatry and psychology are often obscured by the methodological limitations of past research. It is only recently that a handful of studies has been launched which will satisfy the criteria set forth by Sheldon White:

> Program decisions based on manipulating powerful single variables that affect large segments of the population of children are not now derivable from the evidence we reviewed. We do not know enough about human developmental antecedents of particular adult characteristics. Studies of only one variable are not likely to yield predictive relationships. *The one generalization emerging again and again is that all variables and their interactions must be considered simultaneously* (White et al., 1973).

Further criticism is leveled at multivariate techniques, because (1) the variables are conglomerate; (2) there is often poor measurement, which means we are dealing with higher orders of error, thus in more complex models the imprecision is greatly magnified; (3) usually few variables are used in linear relationships; and (4) it is suggested that path analysis is a welcome addition to these techniques (White et al., 1973).

Since a large portion of the variables usually found in child studies has been included in our predictor sets, and multiple regression analysis with all interactions and variables present has been conducted (along with some path analysis still in progress), this report will rank order the variables found in a very scant review of the literature, in terms of the relative contributions to variance in child behaviors found in our study, both concurrently and longitudinally. Those variables not significantly related to child behavior in our study will not be reviewed, to save space.

In the Family Research Project, characteristics of parents and their marriage were factored into eight dimensions, as shown in Table 2−3. The way in which parents related to their children, usually called child rearing and home atmosphere variables, formed five dimensions, as shown in Table 2−4. These were not parental attitudes toward child rearing, nor were they retrospective. They were descriptions of their current behavior toward the child.

These tables show the factors and give brief examples of items from the mother's questionnaire which, during the separate factoring processes, correlated highly with the dimension in question. The reliability of the dimensions is also shown. Most of the relationships between these dimensions were quite low (around .20) because the orthogonal factor model is designed to develop factors that are as independent of one another as possible.

In addition, 45 demographic variables were included, of which only eleven showed significant relationships to child behavior when other factors were included in the equation. These variables will be discussed in approximate order of the number of behaviors they predicted, and of their unique predictive power for behavior—that is, the predictive association that remains when all other variables used in the study were controlled. Note again, we didn't control genetic history, aspects of the physical environment, diet, pre- and perinatal history, and so on; and left out many important variables for such reasons as time, money, lack of skills, lack of instruments, and research bias.

1. Parents Punitive. While this predictor ranked fourth in power in the concurrent relationship to Year I behavior dimensions (see Table 2−5), it was by far the most powerful *long term* predictor to Year V[a] behavior of the child. Our longitudinal study enables us to compare the present power or associative strength and future power or true forecasting power of predictors, and a very different picture emerges.

It is important to know both of these relationships, since prevention and intervention may have both short and long term goals. Punitiveness has more unique contributions to behavior over time, and these were of larger size, than any other familial predictor variable. Especially in the area of aggression and antisocial behavior, the long term contributions were about as large or even greater than its concurrent contributions. It is possible that some of our childhood

[a]The Year V followup interviews were not always five years later than the Year I interviews, due to problems of locating families, etc. The terms Time I and Time II are more accurate.

Table 2–3. The Eight Parental Factors, with Representative Items and Their Factor Loadings and the Reliability Coefficient of the Factor

Factor	Content	Correlation with Factor Score	Reliability Coefficient
1 Isolated Parents (N = 9)[a]	Parents have no close friends or few close friends and have visitors or visit less than once a month	.38	.74
		.34	
2 Unhappy Marriage (N = 10)	Parents say that their marriage is an unhappy one and	.67	.85
	that they are more unhappy than their friends	.60	
3 Mother's Physical and Emotional Illness (N = 11)	Mother's health is poor	.59	.81
	Mother has periods when she can't get going	.54	
	feels weak all over and	.52	
	is often bothered by nervousness	.51	
4 Unleisurely Parents (N = 18)	Parents do not have free time or don't use it for	.50	.83
	music	.49	
	reading	.27	
	arts and handicrafts	.32	
	They do not belong to groups or clubs		
5 Mother's Economic Dissatisfaction (N = 13)	Mother would like to have her own home and other possessions	.46	.68
		.35	

6 Parents' Quarrels ($N = 14$)		.81
Mother is not satisfied with her husband and herself	.51	
Family disagreements are over money	.40	
free time and	.30	
her husband's occupation	.28	
	.25	
7 Husband Ill and Withdrawn—Unaffectionate Marriage ($N = 8$)		.69
The husband is ill and	.41	
does not show affection easily to his wife	.44	
8 Traditional Marriage ($N = 9$)		.66
Being a parent is the most important role for both parents	.42	
Mother attends religious services frequently	.41	

[a] N is the number of items in the factor.

Table 2–4. The Five Parent-Child Factors, with Representative Items and Their Factor Loadings and the Reliability Coefficient of the Factor

Factor	Content	Correlation with Factor Score	Reliability Coefficient
1 Parents Cold (N = 14)[a]	Parents rarely hug and kiss the child or	.43	.77
	show affection easily to the child	.40	
2 Mother Traditional Restrictive (N = 21)	Mother is not informed through books, magazines, or media about children	.71	.88
	She gives bizarre explanations about sex—warns the child about sex	.50	
	She views being "quiet and well-behaved" as important	.27	
3 Parents Punitive (N = 15)	Parents spank child with a strap or stick and	.63	.81
	often use deprivation of privileges	.60	
4 Mother Supportive-Directing (N = 16)	When the child is upset or lonely, the mother tries to cheer him up and distract him	.53	.79
	When the child is rebellious the mother	.42	
	does not try to change him	.45	
	but tries to talk to him about it	.36	
5 Mother Excitable-Rejecting (N = 15)	Mother often screams at child, is very changeable in handling him, and regards	.39	.83
	self as an excitable person when handling	.37	
	child	.31	

[a]N is the number of items in the factor.

predictors have a "sleeper" effect (Stouffer, 1950), in that their concurrent effect is small or even absent in comparison with their long term effect. A delayed effect has been mentioned in connection with the emergence of disturbed heterosexual behavior (shyness or promiscuousness) during the adolescence, but not in the preadolescence, of girls whose fathers were absent earlier (Hetherington and Deur, 1970).

Child abuse is socially undesirable behavior, yet this did not deter 7 percent of the cross-section or 21 percent of the welfare sample mothers from reporting that they beat the child with a stick or strap. While only 25 child abusers were officially reported from our sample by our record search, several hundred children could easily be considered to be in this category. This does not include verbal abuse, or cruel but nonviolent punishment. Stopping child abuse, using group methods for known abusers, and especially discussing punishment with potential parents in high school and during the first pregnancy with fathers present, is a high priority goal for preventing mental disorder in children for both the short and long term. The key idea is that if there was punishment in Year I, even if punishment stops in Year V, there is more likely to be antisocial behavior in the older child. In a sense, then, the effects of the factor are not reversible.

The relationship between both maternal and paternal punishment, and the severity of punishment and aggression has been found in many studies (Rosenthal et al., 1959; Baumrind, 1967; Hetherington, Stouwie & Ridberg, 1970; Sears, Maccoby & Levin, 1957; Sears, Whiting, Nowlis & Sears, 1953; Becker et. al., 1962). Some differences were found between boys and girls. Extremes of the punishment dimension (high and low punishment) were linked to passivity and low assertiveness in girls (Becker, 1962). Girls also showed more aggression-anxiety associated with punishment (Sears, 1961). The absence of punishment was found more frequent in overanxious clinic children (Jenkins, 1968) and punishment was used less than reasoning, rewards, or discussion by mothers of boys with high self-esteem (Baumrind, 1967).

For most studies punishment predicted antisocial behavior, mostly in boys, at home and in school. In our study, however, it did not predict aggression within the home, only outside it. There were no significant interaction effects by age, sex, mother's education, or ethnic background in the Family Research Project Year I data, so that the association of punitiveness with antisocial behavior holds for both sexes in our sample.

A review of longitudinal studies on abuse, neglect and undernourishment (White, 1973) finds the data limited, but shows a high pro-

Table 2–5.   Time I Predictors of Child Behavior at Time I (Concurrent) and at Time II (Long Term or Forecasting), with Percentage of Variance Predicted, in Rank Order of Predictive Power by Time I[a]

Predictor	Behaviors Predicted	% Unique Variance		Totals	
		Time I[a]	Time II	Time I	Time II
Mother Excitable-Rejecting	1. Conflict with parents	8.9	1.0		
	2. Regressive anxiety	4.0			
	3. Fighting	3.8			
	4. Sex curiosity	3.2			
	5. Isolation	2.0			
	6. Self-destructive tendencies	1.9			
	7. Conflict with siblings	1.9			
	8. Mentation problems	1.5			
	9. Competition	1.2			
	10. (Impairment[b] of school functioning)	1.2			
	Total number predicted			9	1
	Average % variance predicted			3.3	1.0
	Predictor rank			1	9
Parents Cold	1. Conflict with parents	7.8	2.6		
	2. Fighting	2.1			
	3. Conflict with siblings	1.5			
	4. Undemanding	1.0			
	5. Delinquency	1.0			
	Total number predicted			5	1
	Average % variance predicted			2.7	2.6
	Predictor rank			2	4
Spanish-speaking	1. Isolation	3.7	2.1		
	2. Weak group membership	2.7			
	3. Mentation problems	1.3			

4. Training difficulties	1.3	1.0		
5. Compulsivity	1.2	1.4		
6. (Less) regressive anxiety		1.3		
7. Dependence		1.0		
8. (Less) conflict with parents[c]				
Total number predicted			5	5
Average % variance predicted			2.0	1.6
Predictor rank			3	1
Parents Punitive				
1. Fighting	2.6	2.3		
2. Conflict with parents	1.9	1.0		
3. Regressive anxiety	1.0			
4. Delinquency		1.4		
Total number predicted			3	3
Average % variance predicted			1.8	1.6
Predictor rank			4	2
Mother's Physical and Emotional Illness				
1. Regressive anxiety	2.1	2.1		
2. Fighting	1.1			
Total number predicted			2	1
Average % variance predicted			1.7	2.1
Predictor rank			5	6
Black				
1. Mentation problems	1.8			
2. Demandingness	1.1			
3. (Impairment[b] of school functioning)	1.3			
4. Dependence		1.3		
5. (Less) conflict with parents[c]		1.1		
6. Repetitive motor behavior		1.0		
Total number predicted			2	3
Average % variance predicted			1.5	1.1
Predictor rank			6	3

(*Table 2-5. continued overleaf*)

Table 2–5. continued

Predictor	Behaviors Predicted	% Unique Variance		Totals	
		Time I[a]	Time II	Time I	Time II
High Number of Addresses	1. Delinquency	1.4			
	2. Fighting	1.2			
	3. (Impairment of school functioning)	1.2			
	Total number predicted			2	0
	Average % variance predicted			1.3	0.0
	Predictor rank			7	10
High Rent	1. Conflict with parents	1.2			
	2. Isolation	1.0			
	3. (Less) dependence		1.1		
	Total number predicted			2	1
	Average % variance predicted			1.1	1.1
	Predictor rank			8	8
Large Number of Children in the Household	1. (Less) competition	1.2			
	2. (Impairment of school functioning)	1.2			
	3. Regressive anxiety		1.6		
	Total number predicted			1	1
	Average % variance predicted			1.2	1.6
	Predictor rank			9	7
Number of Natural Parents	1. Delinquency	1.0			
	Total number predicted			1	0
	Average % variance predicted			1.0	0.0
	Predictor rank			10	11

Table 2–5. continued

Predictor	Behaviors Predicted	% Unique Variance		Totals	
		Time I[a]	Time II	Time I	Time II
Mother Traditional Restrictive[d]	1. Dependence		2.5		
	Total number predicted			0	1
	Average % variance predicted			0.0	2.5
	Predictor rank			11	5

[a] Using criterion of a minimum of 1% unique variance for inclusion.

[b] Impairment areas were not included, as they were not rated at Time II except for Total Impairment. However, impairment of school and thus cognitive functioning seemed too important to leave out. It was not included in the ranking.

[c] Since being Spanish or Black predicted less Conflict with Parents, being White predicted more.

[d] To simplify presentation, four weak concurrent predictors have been deleted; Traditional marriage, Mother's economic dissatisfaction, Unleisurely parents, and Parents quarrels.

portion of serious outcomes, such as brain injury, mental retardation, permanent physical injury, and emotional problems. Our review and own findings point to the emotional problems being primarily aggressive and antisocial behavior.

2. Mother Excitable-Rejecting. This predictor is a combination of mother's excitability (screaming) and changeability. It partakes of the parental "aggressiveness" and "inconsistency" variables common in the literature. While most studies have found it associated with conduct disorders and antisocial behavior, we found it was concurrently correlated with self-destructiveness, mentation problems, anxiety, and isolation, as well as with fighting and conflict with both parents and siblings, among others. However, it was not related to delinquency except in the welfare families.

It was associated with 19 behaviors or impairment ratings in Year I, the largest number of associations for any predictor. Interestingly, the long term predictive power for this factor fell to one-tenth of its concurrent power. This means that there is some long term effect for Year I excitability of mothers, but not a great deal. However, this is a tremendously important element in the child's immediate environment, and should be taken into account for short term effects on almost all behavior.

It would seem worthwhile to recommend desensitization for the intense emotionality and anger in mothers, preventive programs to educate prospective mothers, or even high school baby sitters, in a set of coping skills with children. The damage that may result from highly charged emotionality such as screaming, and from being inconsistent or changeable, should be communicated early before initial damage is done. Having a husband, or having any other adult in the household, may be a large factor in calming mothers. Kellam, in his analysis of family composition and its effects in an assessment and intervention program (Kellam and Schiff, 1967 and subsequent papers), found that the myriad family types did not discriminate, but mother alone versus mother with husband or anyone else did discriminate between levels of adjustment and types of children.

In many studies, aggressive or excitable parents predicted to conduct disorders, delinquency, or aggressiveness. Several studies found there was evidence for modeling of aggressive parents by their children (Bandura & Walters, 1963; Berkowitz, 1962; Becker, 1959). Some studies found inconsistency of one parent (Rosenthal et al., 1959), or inconsistency between parents (Baruch & Wilcox, 1944), or one restrictive and one lax parent, typically the mother (Read, 1945), leading to maladjustment or antisocial behavior. Erratic control by mothers was found in aggressive boys (McCord, McCord & Howard, 1961), and inconsistent, lax, or erratic discipline by both parents was found in delinquent boys (Andry, 1960; Bandura & Walters, 1959; Burt, 1929; Glueck and Glueck, 1950; McCord et al., 1959; and Merrill, 1947).

There is some evidence that consistency, whether warm or cold, is helpful to the child in providing the well known "stable set of expectations," which often turn out to be Augean. The type of predictor that could be considered either social in nature (based upon modeling) or genetic is the criminality of family members. A background of criminality was found in 84 percent of delinquents in a Massachusetts reformatory (Glueck & Glueck, 1950), and was found by others to be associated with a high incidence of antisocial behavior (Shaw and McKay, 1942). The preponderance of associations with delinquency in the literature, in contrast to the wide range of associations between excitable parents and various child behaviors in our random sample using a prospective design, may indicate the type of oversight possible when studying known groups of apprehended or treated children or adults retrospectively or in a follow-back design.

3. **Parental Coldness.** This factor was linked significantly to five behaviors in Year I, which were expressive of conflict with parents, peers, siblings and the larger community. Children with cold parents were also undemanding, which is also more common in older children. However, one eventually does not demand what one cannot get. Conversely, parents may not respond to a child who is undemanding. This factor also had a predictive power that was only one-tenth as great as its concurrent power. Here the literature shows a wider range of associated behaviors than our study.

There is a problem of including hostility as the extreme end of the warmth-coldness dimension. In our study, rejection, punishment, and coldness were independent factors, which may account for the more limited range of associations we found. While rejection and hostility, especially by father, were found in delinquent boys (Andry, 1960; Bandura & Walters, 1959; Glueck & Glueck, 1950; McCord et. al., 1959; Merrill, 1947), retardation, depression, withdrawal, psychosomatic disorders, and neurosis were all linked with aspects of coldness. Maternal hostility, which may not be coldness, was negatively correlated with intelligence tests 30 years later, and early maternal affection correlated positively with intelligence in middle age (Bayley, 1968).

Retarded girls made emotional and intellectual progress when "adopted" by older retarded girls (Skeels, 1967). Cold and impersonal handling and maternal deprivation have been indicted in many studies often associated with wasting syndrome or extreme withdrawal (Spitz, 1946; Bower, Shellhamer & Dailey, 1960; Bowlby & Ainsworth, 1964). Schaefer (1961, 1959) identified love vs. hostility as part of the circumplex model of maternal behavior, which was mentioned as a problem since our factor structure seemed to separate coldness and hostility, the latter usually inferred by aggression toward the child. Little affection, attention, or stimulation was found associated with depression and withdrawal in intact families (Coleman & Provence, 1957) as well as in institutional settings. This makes us more confident that cold handling, whether in patient populations or in the family, is producing the effects. While little closeness was observed between mothers and children who were normal, psychosomatic, or neurotic, the mothers of severely disturbed children were completely oblivious and impervious to them (Garner & Wenar, 1959).

These findings could be documented by myriad studies of animals as well as humans. There is no evidence of relationships between coldness and anxiety or depression in our data. This makes one wonder if marasmus or withdrawal is more often found in infant studies of institutionalization, while the evidence for antisocial behavior is strong in older children, where it is of course more likely to occur. Since our sample starts at age 6, the more helpless reactions to parental coldness may be minimized.

4. Mother's Physical and Emotional Illness. This could indeed be the predictor closest to suggesting a genetic connection between mother's disturbance and children's disturbance. The factor was related to two child behaviors concurrently but had, like most of the other factors we'll mention from now on, little long term predictive power. The questions on this dimension are mainly from a screening instrument associated with adult impairment of role function based on the Midtown Manhattan Study (Langner, 1962) and are mostly psychophysiological in nature.

Unique contributions of Mother's Emotional Illness were to anxiety in her child, to fighting, and to a larger dimension made of these and depression-like symptoms such as crying. The hypothesis that modeling is involved is less tenable for fighting behavior than for anxiety, since the mothers do not evidence fighting (at least the mother's symptom items only measure depression, anxiety, somatization, and possible physical illness). The pattern of child behaviors and their rank order is very different from that of other predictors.

For this reason there is less likelihood of mere circularity, in that a sick mother reports a sick child.

In the literature, neurotic adults and neurotic children are more likely to come from parents with neurotic symptoms (Bennett, 1960; Jenkins, 1966; Shields & Slater, 1961). Children referred to a child guidance clinic had parents with more deviant MMPI profiles (Liverant, 1959). Looking at the opposite side of the mental health-disorder continuum, boys with high self-esteem had mothers with high self-esteem, who were satisfied with their husbands and had low conflict with them (Baumrind, 1967). Data on mental hospitalization showed little relation to children's behavior, but our data were self-reported and not based upon a record search. Given that much mental disorder goes untreated, it is possible that the low association between treatment and impairment is responsible for this negative finding.

Any program for children should treat both parent and child. While we neglected father's mental health (since we felt that the mother could not report his symptoms for him), there is every reason to view both parents as necessary participants in preventive or therapeutic programs. School preparatory programs that don't continue to use the parents to reinforce the early positive behavior may fail. It is unfortunate that more detailed assessment of the mother's symptoms was not undertaken in Time I, but this has been expanded at Time II, and has yet to be explored in detail, to see if mother's depersonalization, immobilization, depressed mood, and somatization are differentially associated with child behavior.

5, 6. **Race—Ethnic Background and Social Class.** These predictors are discussed together because there is a general feeling that they are closely interrelated. This overlap does not mean that they are not capable of making independent contributions to adult and child behavior. Bruce Dohrenwend, in his paper on the genesis of mental disorders (Dohrenwend, 1975), has said that before we study the interactions between genetic predisposition and environmental stress in producing disorder, we should "move from the vivid bodies of descriptive data that have accumulated on relations between sociocultural and social-psychological factors and psychopathology toward new research aimed at demonstrating which if any of these factors are important in etiology."

We could not agree more with this statement, but we think an excellent strategy for weeding out the freeloading factors and establishing causal sequences is the use of multiple regression and path analysis, techniques which we already have. His ingenious reanalysis of Robins' data showed that blacks have over four times the rate of antisocial personality of whites within the low socioeconomic status group, and in so doing demonstrated that sociocultural factors are important in etiology. However, the samples are small, and the actual associative and true predictive power of the relationship, as opposed to its statistical significance, was not clear. Race and class are not placed in simultaneous context with other environmental factors, so we don't know their strength relative to other aspects of the environment. Most frustrating for all researchers is the conglomerate nature of these large rubrics, which must be "psychologized," in a positive sense of the term, to show how they or their component variables produce their effects.

The level of complexity of the variables chosen is a major deterrent to further understanding. More social-psychological constructs need to be brought into studies *before* they go into the field to explain why there are connections between demographic predictors and disorder. Let's briefly take some examples from Dr. Dohrenwend's current paper on adult disorders (Dohrenwend, 1976). Consistently over many total prevalence studies, women show more neurosis (perhaps neurotic depressions?) and more manic-depressive psychoses than men, while men exhibit more personality disorders and antisocial behavior. Why is this so? As an example of a predictor of a lower order of generality than sex, we can consider self-esteem.

A community in Mexico which was known historically for the high self-esteem, prestige, and equality of its women was contrasted with more traditional Mexico City. Women with high self-esteem and pro-feminine attitudes were found to have much lower rates of reported symptoms than their low-esteem peers, in relation to the symptom levels of the men in their own communities (Langner, 1965). The anxious-depressed-somatizing dimension which is tapped by the symptom checklist fits in with the neurotic-depressed dimension found to differ by sex in so many studies. However, it is not being a woman, but being a person of low self-esteem, that seems to account for much of the variance. Similar low-esteem groups, such as minorities, the unemployed, and lower class groups, should be linked to depression in a series of studies that include depression and other scales of disorder to make sure of the specificity of the relationship. Random samples that include these and a full range of demographic and other predictors should be included.

Differential child rearing practices are another etiological factor. It has been observed that some mothers will for long periods braid, brush, or comb the hair of a physically active daughter starting just at the point the girl initiates physical activity, such as running or jumping. If such observations can be made reliably, contrasting boys and girls, and followed up, the frequency and length of restraint procedures may predict quiet-depressed disorders versus active disorders such as antisocial behavior.

As women's status in our society grows, can we expect more evidence of socialized antisocial behavior in women? Leighton found more sociopathic and less psychoneurotic behavior in women in some socially "disintegrated areas" (Leighton, et al., 1963) than in women in other parts of Stirling County. "Both quantitatively and qualitatively they present a picture similar to that of the men." There was previous evidence that twice as many mothers in the Disintegrated Area, in contrast to cohesive communities, believe there is no difference between "masculine" and "feminine" behavior (Hughes et al., 1960).

Similar variables can be employed, and have been employed, to study the effect of social class upon disorders. If there is consistently more disorder at lower class levels, especially schizophrenia and personality disorder, then we must ask why. Is it preselection by downward drift? (Jarvis, 1971). This might seem supported by the fact that schizophrenics show seclusiveness from an early age (Clausen & Kohn, 1960). However, our own study points out that as much as a fifth of the general child population shows seclusive and isolative behavior. What we see retrospectively from patient studies is again misleading, since prospectively, only a tiny fraction of these seclusive children will ever become schizoid or schizophrenic.

Is the association caused by living in socially disorganized areas of cities (Faris and Dunham, 1939)? We can again ask more specific questions, depending on our training and skills. Is there parental modeling for schizophrenia and antisocial behavior? There is some evidence for this (Rosenthal, 1974). Even in careful studies of adoption of children of schizophrenic mothers at birth, there are flaws, such as the fact that by law in some states the adoptive parent must know that the mother was in a mental hospital. The overanxious or overprotective behavior of such an adoptive parent or relative may constitute a special learning situation for the child, which contributes beyond the genetic risk (Heston, 1966). Information about the mother's schizophrenia may be transmitted directly to the child and to teachers and peers, with the effects on the child's behavior coming in good part from the social stigma. Social scientists and genetically oriented clinicians should learn some of each other's skills in order to be aware of the pitfalls of their designs.

Other predictors might be measures of the double-bind hypothesis such as the conflict and dominance measures of the Revealed Difference Test (Farina, 1960). Family members are asked individually how they would handle a series of child-rearing problems if alone. The family is then brought together to discuss and solve each problem. Conflict measures include frequency of simultaneous speech, interruptions, disagreements and aggressions, failure to reach agreement, and total speaking time. These are non-inferential, and highly reliable measures. This sounds fine, but to use it with families of childhood schizophrenics has at least two major design flaws: (1) the presence of conflicting signals must be established *before* the onset of the disorder if they are to be considered causal; and (2) there is little continuity between childhood autism, atypical development, childhood schizophrenia, and the adult forms which occur from the early 20s on.

One solution, fanciful in view of the current cutbacks in funding, but a hope for the future, would be a gigantic prospective study of 100,000 people, starting from birth, or at marriage of the parents, with complete records, consistent medical care and examination, and periodic screening and observation in multiple settings. A small percentage, say 5000 people, could be set aside for different preventive and treatment modalities to be applied on a random basis. Measures for all the major suspected etiological factors in mental disorder would be gathered or created, and the research team would have weekly electrocardiograms, to insure continuity of method. With a large enough sample, a prospective study including even rare disorders is possible. With the advent of changes in the funding of medical care, this type of womb to tomb study may be possible.

A massive longitudinal study of 11,000 children in England (Kellmer-Pringle, Butler & Davie, 1966 and Gooch & Kellmer-Pringle, 1966), where such sizeable studies have in the past been more possible to conduct, has reported on children's symptoms. Low socioeconomic status was found to be associated with high maladjustment. Unfortunately, none of the more specific explanatory variables were gathered, but differential child rearing is hypothesized as the causal factor. While the descriptive data in a study of this size are excellent, the etiological leads are slim, stopping again at the demographic level of understanding. In sum, more explanatory measures, such as family cohesion, warmth, disparagement, permissiveness for agression outside the home, self esteem, vertical mobility and reasons for moving, and changes in any of these measures, might be helpful in tracing the sources of antisocial and schizophrenic disorders.

The social learning approach need not deal only with external behavior. It can deal with internal behaviors without invoking unconscious mechanisms, yet not ignore them if they seem to help in an explanatory chain, and can be objectified and measured in some consistent way. Self-image, aspiration level, model internalization, degree of bonding to others, are all intervening explanatory variables or concepts which can be measured, and are in a middle range between demographic rubrics and individual microdynamics.

There are not many total prevalence studies of behavior disorder in children. Most of those that exist are excellent studies, with the usual limitations imposed by time, funding, personal skills, and the state of the art. While not exhaustive, the following are major studies focusing on child symptoms of psychiatric significance: MacFarlane, Allen & Honzik (1954) studied 252 children, followed for fourteen years, using mother's reports. The subjects were a random sample of Berkeley, California, of fairly high SES, all white. One half were controls, others in guidance. Lapouse and Monk (1958) studied a random sample of 482 children in Buffalo, New York, using mother's reports, and a 10 percent sample of children self-reported. Robins' (1966) study has been described previously. It is a follow-back design to 524 persons seen as children in the St. Louis Municipal Psychiatric Clinic, plus matched controls.

Thomas, Chess & Birch (1968) followed 136 normal babies from birth, using observation and parent interviews. By age 9, 42 were given psychiatric care. Nine behavioral or temperamental attributes scored in infancy were unrelated to pathology except high activity level in Year 1, and high intensity in Year 3. Some evidence of the interaction between temperament and parental behavior was seen as productive of the disorders. Douglas studied 5362 children born in one week of 1946 in England and Wales, and they were followed to age 20 (Douglas 1964, 1966; Mulligan et al., 1963). In this study, with class "controlled," families of delinquents had more inadequate parents than families of non-delinquents. (Inadequate meant less educated, more quarrelsome, more often separated, or making less use of health services.) This is suggestive that not class, but parental behavior, is more important for delinquency. This seems affirmed in our data. Robins and Lewis (1966) found antisocial (inadequate?) parents or grandparents increased the risk of a son's dropping out of high school or getting a police or juvenile court record, in *both* white collar and blue collar families.

Tuddenham, Brooks, and Milkovich (1974) had mothers sort cards containing a behavior inventory of 100 items into "True," "Not True" and "Uncertain" categories. These descriptions applied to their 3049 children aged 9 to 11. While largely middle class due to membership in the Kaiser Health Plan in Oakland, California, there was an adequate proportion of black children, 21 percent, to afford stable comparative figures, as well as smaller proportions of Orientals and Chicanos (about 4 and 3 percent respectively). Frequency data on the 100 items were reported by sex and ethnic group, and by mother's education. There were many significant differences for individual symptoms found according to these variables, but their relative strengths are difficult to assess. There was a decreasing prevalence of about 1/10 of the items with increasing mother's educational level, but primarily among white children.

The authors suggest that children of better educated mothers are both more socialized and more secure, or that these mothers may be less critical of their children's behavior. Our results do not show mother's education making an independent contribution to child behavior, but acting as a mediating variable in many relationships, especially in parental behavior toward the child. Tuddenham, Brooks, and Milkovich compare their results with similar studies, including Glidewell (1968), Lapouse and Monk (1958, 1964), Long (1941), MacFarlane et al. (1954), the National Health Survey (1971), and two British studies, Rutter, Tizard & Whitmore (1970), and Shepherd et al. (1971). These surveys are all recommended for further study.

The results closely parallel those of Tuddenham et al. The major difficulty is that symptoms are usually only treated individually. This makes for unreliability, since they are only single representatives of dimensions of behavior. In addition, while some variables are controlled for class or race, the relative contributions of each are not measured. Tests of significance are the primary statistical tool. A reanalysis of these studies to determine the simultaneous concurrent power of the predictors would be very helpful.

In the Family Research Project, unique contributions of ethnic background and race constitute the third most powerful concurrent predictor after the parent-child factors. Being Spanish-speaking (compared with other ethnic groups) is linked with five behavior scores, accounting for from 3.7 to 1.2 percent variance. These include Isolation, Weak Group Membership, Training Problems, Mentation Problems, and Compulsivity. Being black accounted for variance in two scores, ranging from 1.8 to 1.1 percent, including Mentation Problems, and Demandingness.

In addition to these concurrent relationships, ethnic background has the greatest forecasting power of any variable if considered as a group (see Table 2−5). Being Spanish-speaking at Time I forecast being Dependent and having Weak Group Membership at Time II. Being non-Spanish-speaking forecast being non-Compulsive (or mildly antisocial) and being Anxious. Being black at Time I forecast being Dependent or exhibiting Repetitive Motor Behavior, such as spinning, toe-walking, head-banging, etc. Being white forecast greater Conflict with Parents. These behaviors in children now averaging five years older are less prevalent, less age-appropriate, and more serious in their implications. Ethnic background forecasts eight types of behavior, with a range of from 1 to 2.1 percent variance accounted for.

Of all predictors, only having Punitive Parents rivals this long term predictivity, being related to three behaviors; Fighting, Delinquency, and Conflict with Parents, with a range of 1 to 2.3 percent of variance accounted for. Such weights make the selection of high risk groups relatively easy, and can facilitate sample selection for related research. Excitable Mothers, Cold Parents, Mother's Emotional Illness, low Rent and a small Number of Children were related over time either to the same behaviors they were originally associated with at Time I, or they mirrored those relationships in some way. However, mother's being Traditional-Restrictive forecast Dependency, bringing in a new predictor which had not had any concurrent strength (except in the Welfare sample).

A step from associations toward causal explanations lies in the analysis of change. The standardized regressed change score tells us if a person's percentile standing on a dimension has changed over time when the effects of "regression toward the mean" have been controlled. If parents become warmer, or less rejecting, this was significantly associated with improvements in, (or less of) Conflict with Parents, Regressive Anxiety, Fighting, Mentation Problems, Isolation, and Delinquency. These relationships could also be stated in the reverse causal sequence; for example, a lessening of psychopathology in the children on these dimensions produced a corresponding improvement in the behavior of the parents toward the child.

We are now attempting to compare groups of parents and children who exhibit more or less severe parenting and more or less severe pathology at both Time I and Time II, or at one time but not the other. By this method we may be able to establish the time sequence between parental and child behavior. For example, a group of families in which parents did not exhibit severe parenting at Time I, but did at Time II, should show children with predominantly increasing levels of behavior pathology, not with continuous levels. The length of exposure of the child to parental behavior may become a critical factor. Changes seem consistent with theories of role model behavior, and thus with parental behavior being primary. Changes in Parental Coldness and Excitability were tied to changes in aggressive behavior in all settings. Changes in Parental Punitiveness were only related to changes in intrafamilial aggression, but not aggression toward peers or society in general.

The question is whether physical punishment in particular serves as a model for much later behavior in settings where aggression may be rewarded more than it is within the family. Coldness and excitability, in contrast, might operate through producing frustration, and hence concurrent, not delayed, aggression rather than through imitation or role modeling behavior.

One percent of variance equals a partial correlation of .10. The percent of variance equals the square of the correlation. Thus the range of correlations we are talking about runs from .10, or 1 percent variance, the arbitrary lower limit for discussion, to .32, or 10 percent variance. While these may seem small, they are unique contributions or partial correlations, taking out the effect of as many as twenty five other factors simultaneously, so only the portion of child behavior which is accounted for by this variable alone (excluding factors not in the equation) shows in the percentage. Multiple correlations for some behavior run as high as 45 percent at Time I (a correlation of .67), and when Time II predictors are added, as high as 60 percent, or a multiple correlation of .78.

Taking all the environment we have tried to measure, with inevitably imprecise yardsticks, we can account for 60 percent of the variation in some child behaviors measured at Time II. This is good, especially when one considers that such factors as genetic history, degree of racial discrimination, physical measurements and blood parameters, neighborhood characteristics, air and noise pollution level, and many other factors have been left out. The addition of changes in variables as predictors may increase the proportion of disorder variance predicted. The contribution of any one of 25 factors will not be large, but it represents its actual power relative to the other variables in the whole set, and quantification is what is crucial at this point, along with some answers to the "why" questions. The mere addition of new predictors may obscure the picture, since after a point there is a great deal of overlap between them, and the new factors may not add to the prediction.

In a previous paper, a breakdown of the components of being black, white, or Spanish-speaking showed that the amount of stress, not in terms of events as much as in terms of processes or relationships, could account for the different levels of disorder by race (Langner, Gersten & Eisenberg, 1974). How cold, punitive, or excitable were parents of these groups? How unhappy were their marriages, how much emotional illness did the mothers in these groups exhibit? How many children were in their families, how often had they moved, were their mothers caring for the children? The stress rankings coincided with the ranking of blacks and Spanish-speaking having more impaired children. It did not rank the minorities exactly, since their children were very close in overall behavior scores, but the black stress scores were higher than the Spanish stress scores.

Roughly speaking, the distribution of stresses or predictors by ethnic background accounted for the white vs. minority difference in disorder rates. This tells us two things; first that one can psychologize or sociologize demographic conglomerates and get results, and second, that race still accounts for something in its own right which we haven't eliminated, but this might more likely be exposure to prejudice, poor diet, or low birth weight, than it might be some genetic contribution.

In contrast, race variables contributed concurrently more than class variables to two large groups of behavior variables out of three. These were Organic-Developmental symptoms and Delinquency. Only the large group Anxiety-Depression was predicted better by class than by race (Langner, Gersten & Eisenberg, 1974). In true forecasting, race or ethnic variables were even more powerful in relation to other factors than they were concurrently. They were the highest ranking prognostic factors. The belief that class controls will wash out ethnic contributions must be re-examined.

7. Other Predictors. Space considerations preclude more detailed consideration of the remaining predictors which did account for child behavior, and of those which did not. A listing (in Table 2−5) shows that Moving a great deal, perhaps as a result of uprooting, was related to Fighting and Delinquency. High Rent was linked to conflict with parents and siblings, perhaps mostly a reflection of a middle class atmosphere permissive for intrafamilial expression of anger. A large Number of Children in the Household was related to reduced competition and impairment of the children's school functioning. While other impairment ratings were not discussed, this particular relationship has appeared in the literature, and seems important.

Reduced family size, through birth control, would probably improve overall school performance. The amount of time even middle class parents spend with younger children in their large families is limited inevitably by their number. The children also tend to form a relatively noncompetitive peer group. "Number of natural parents," or broken homes, consists mostly of absent fathers. This we found associated with delinquency only, and there are many corroborations in the literature (Bacon, Child & Barry 1963; Biller 1970; Glueck & Glueck 1950).

However, the lack of association with other behaviors in our data is of special interest, since neurotic problems such as anxiety and depression, and homosexuality, are believed to stem from absent fathers, or early death of fathers, as well. These findings may be the result of starting with patient groups. Generally, investigators have found that conditions leading up to parental absence, such as parental conflict, are more important than the event itself, and the quality of family life before and after separation is critical (White et al., 1973). Mother absence is really not represented in our study since there were relatively few cases in which the mother was not present.

Prevention and Intervention

Putting these predictors into family profile types has helped us to better understand their relationships. Short of a presentation of these types, it would seem best to recommend that prevention concentrate on the specific factors mentioned, though family types can be high risk groups. At this point it would be helpful to review very briefly the major predictors which become points or leads for prevention and intervention. Table 2–6 places them in rank order of predictive power by averaging both short term (concurrent) and long term (forecasting) power. The number of the eighteen child behaviors associated with each predictor, and the average of the percentage of variance predicted produced a rank for each "Time." These two ranks were then averaged.

The highest ranking predictors are being Spanish-speaking, having Punitive Parents, or Cold Parents, being Black, and having an Excitable-Rejecting Mother. What can be done about this list of devils? How can they be cast out? Physical punishment must be stopped or mitigated. Child beating is almost unheard of in some cultures, so it must be amenable to social intervention by legal strictures and by the creation of an atmosphere condemning it. Coldness is perhaps more difficult to change, but often going through the motions of hugging and kissing a child can eventually stimulate a parent to develop more real warmth. Not only conditioning, but discussion of parental behavior and its origins is helpful, and possibly not too expensive in group form through PTA's and pregnancy classes. Similarly, the excitable mother can be exposed to behavior therapy, and group reinforcement will help, especially if mother-child pairs with similar problems are brought into the group.

If screaming, punching, and strapping are made socially undesirable, a deep understanding of their origins in parents may not be necessary. At present, parents in this country feel they have free license to beat their children, just the way teachers did until a law was passed. Birth control is rapidly reducing family size, and the number of unwanted children, which is usually estimated as the

Table 2–6.   Final Rank Order of Predictors, by Sum of Concurrent and Forecasting Ranks

Final Rank	Predictor	Concurrent Time I	Ranks Forecasting Time II	Sum of Ranks
1	Spanish-speaking	3	1	4
2	Parents Punitive	4	2	6
3	Parents Cold	2	4	6
4	Black	6	3	9
5	Mother Excitable-Rejecting	1	9	10
6	Mother's Physical and Emotional Illness	5	6	11
7	Large Number of Children in Household	9	7	16
8	High Rent	8	8	16
9	Mother Traditional-Restrictive	11	5	16
10	High Number of Addresses	7	10	17
11	Number of Natural Parents (mostly father absent)	10	11	21

fourth child or over. Bulldozing of neighborhoods should be minimized, since it is the poorest who must move before the blade, and
it is their children who lose friends while facing new schools and
unfamiliar surroundings. Rehabilitation of dwellings and neighborhoods, when possible, may alleviate this factor.

Loss of parents, particularly fathers, is due primarily to divorce,
abandonment, and separation. Support for marriage via employment,
counseling, and particularly changes in the Welfare system, could
reduce the major portion of broken homes. A small but important
5 percent of the mothers were widows. This is a function of violence,
accidents, and poor physical health. Better health care and occupational safety measures might reduce this predictor. In turn, this might
be able to reduce delinquency, which is its primary associated behavior. What can be said about the higher risks of black and Puerto
Rican children? What is left of the race-and-ethnic variable can be
part diet, part parasitic infestation[b] and many other things, but most
of all it is likely to be discrimination, and the low self-esteem that
goes with it.

With such formidable problems to solve, the clinical psychiatrist
and the behavioral scientist need to divert part of their attention
from rare but interesting disorders to the massive problems of depression, antisocial behavior, severe anxiety, and isolated and backward
children. But you say, why cure warts? Surely these are problems
that pass in time? Contrariwise, they don't always get better with
advancing age, especially problems of antisocial behavior. And while
children in New York City are getting good services relative to the
rest of the country and perhaps the world, *only half the severely
impaired children in our sample were ever referred to any type of
service*, such as a school counsellor, social worker, child psychologist,
or psychiatrist. Only one in five received "long term" treatment of
six months or longer.

Of severely impaired cross-section children, 19 percent got long
term and 30 percent got short term treatment (usually about 1 or 2
visits), while the remaining 51 percent were never seen. Impaired
Welfare children got slightly less treatment; 15 percent long term,
26 percent short term, and 59 percent were never seen. This is not
bad, until you remember that they were *all* severely impaired. For

[b]The Health Research Council of the City of New York reported in 1968
(*Newsletter* Vol. II, No. 1, 5/68) that "New York City's quarter-million Puerto
Rican school-agers have a high incidence of parasitic infections: trichuris or
whipworm 40 percent, amebic infection 30 percent, ascarides or roundworm
18 percent, hookworm 15 percent, strongyloides 15 percent, schistosomiasis 10
percent. Added to dietary deficiencies these worm loads can *stunt a child's
growth*, cause life-long *impairment*."

example, 13.5 percent of the cross-section children, or about one child in seven in Manhattan, were rated by psychiatrists as severely impaired (rated 4 or 5 on a five-point scale). This calls for prevention, not just conventional treatment.

Nationally, about one-third of referrals to child clinics ever get treatment (National Institute of Mental Health, 1966). In our study, the long term treatment group constitutes 35 percent of all those who ever were referred or went for help, almost exactly the national figure. In another survey, only 7 percent got full treatment in typical child guidance clinics, after one fourth quit during intake, 39 percent were referred elsewhere, 11 percent refused treatment after it was offered and 19 percent entered treatment but quit (Hunt, 1961). The problems are clearly in both the family and the services.

Again these figures are deceiving; for British children from a random sample of 6000 who were used as untreated controls matched for symptom severity to a group of clinic children were found to show almost identical improvement rates: 62 percent improved, 29 percent unchanged, and 10 percent worse for the untreated group; and 65 percent improved, 18 percent unchanged, and 16 percent worse in the treated group (Shepherd, Oppenheim, and Mitchell, 1971). This is similar to improvement rates in other child studies, without matched controls. However, children who received five or fewer visits benefited most, regardless of severity of impairment. The preponderance of a few visits as a treatment course may not be, in fact, a tragedy. All this is uncommon sense, and of course needs to be fed into our treatment system as new data come out. Our own tests of treatment effects over five years have not been completed.

In a current analysis, the means on sixteen behavior dimensions show no improvement for children who have been treated over those who have not been treated, holding constant the child's position on three major dimensions of anxiety-depression, organic-developmental problems, and delinquency. A further finding is that children with long term treatment show greater mean pathology on many of the dimensions than those who received short term treatment of six months or more! The findings of Shepherd, Oppenheim, and Mitchell (1971) in Britain seem to be confirmed in our country, at least in this instance. Is it possible that a few visits with some supportive and skilled person with authority tends to help the family mobilize itself, but without self-mobilization there will be deterioration or lack of improvement? The argument that the sicker children and families need more intervention and thus show less progress seems out of keeping with the controls for severity in the British study, and for severity and type of disorder in ours.

In our preliminary work (Gersten et al., 1975) it was assumed that all treated children also improved. Of the initially seriously impaired children, only one-third remained at that level after five years. Of those who improved, only 1 in 25 did so spontaneously (without treatment). Further analysis will show to what degree treatment was actually responsible. No seriously impaired child became well (a rating of 1). Fourteen children per 1000 are being added to the seriously impaired group over five years, vs. only 5.8 per 1000 added to the well–minimally impaired group from other levels. The 14 per 1000 over five years is 2.8 per year per thousand. This true incidence rate describes those children who were not rated 4 or 5 in Year I, but did deteriorate to that level. This is about 2/3 of the rate of 4/1000 for the incidence of myocardial infarction, which has been termed an "epidemic." In absolute numbers, about 4500 children per year aged 6 to 18 become new seriously impaired "cases" in New York City.

There are many suggestions which might be offered for prevention and intervention, which derive directly from some of our seemingly most impractical data. For example, the time at which treatment programs should start is when the behavior syndrome which they are treating is stable enough over time that it does not remit spontaneously in a large portion of the general population. Stability curves for six age cohorts were drawn, using only six child behaviors which were highly correlated with psychiatric impairment ratings (Gersten et al., 1976). Stability coefficients (over the five years) were greater than .55 for five of the six behaviors. Regressive Anxiety, the dimension closest to neurotic disorder, is outgrown up to middle adolescence. Continuity started in middle adolescence, at which time intervention would be more appropriate. Treatment for delinquent-antisocial behavior seems appropriate only at or after preadolescence. Intervention for conduct disorders which involve aggression toward family or peers (Fighting), or speech and thought disturbances (Mentation) should start before age six.

If we know that children generally recover spontaneously from a particular disorder or behavior pattern up to a certain age, it is very wasteful to spend time treating it. Delinquent-antisocial behavior is peer-socialized behavior—unlike fighting at home, which starts much earlier. Recognition of these patterns and their specific times of consolidation or crystallization should allow us to tackle them just before they get entrenched, and at a time when one can definitely no longer say "He'll get over it—it's just a stage."

Barriers to Prevention

The high rate of incidence, and very high rate of prevalence of severe behavioral impairment, urges us to take preventive steps. How can we start new programs when we don't have the personnel and money to take care of the children who need help now? The answer is not to recruit children into traditional programs, but to try to establish very different programs. If one child in seven is severely impaired in a typical urban population, can our society stand this terrible waste? The ultimate and least expensive preventive measure is cutting down on the number of children by contraception and abortion on demand. After that costs can go up to between $13,000 and $36,000 a year per child, often just for custodial care![c] We are now giving real help to only 20 percent of the most severely impaired children, and clinics all have waiting lists.

Do professionals like ourselves really want to see massive change, great new programs of re-education, housing, employment, counselling, legal aid, inexpensive medical care? Except for a few of us, our children go to private schools, we drive to work avoiding the dangerous subways, and many of us live in suburban areas and commute to work. We see the large cities in the United States dying. This is not due to lack of psychiatric facilities, as any Certified Public Accountant will tell you. Is our inaction because of lack of power, or because politics is not our field of specialization? Perhaps for both reasons. Yet there are also great inhibitions to action for the researcher and clinician. After all, to put it bluntly, we thrive on pathology, be it social pathology or lesions of the flesh. Just like the papers, good news doesn't sell. There is no national institute of happiness, but of disease: cancer, drugs and alcohol, heart and lung. Only the National Institute of Mental Health sounds at all positive and happy, and we know that's a coverup: it's really all about schizophrenia and depression.

Kessler & Albee (1975) deal with two barriers to primary prevention. One is the threat to the status quo, since real prevention must make major changes in the social system. The other is the high value we place on privacy and personal freedom of choice as a society, which does not allow us to dictate to others what is "good for them." I quote their most discerning and therefore most irritating comment on the threat of social change.

> To get really involved in primary prevention of emotional disturbance often suggests social and political change quite far removed from the conventional conservatism characteristic of middle class professionals.

[c]Based on figures from Special Services for Children in New York City, 1976, from $35 per day for group homes of twelve children, to over $100 per day in a large institution.

They go on to say that professionals who work with mental patients understand most about the connections between social problems and mental disorder, but because of training are selected to be conscience-laden conservative-to-liberal change agents. Since they are most informed, they are concerned about individual rights. Perhaps this is a double-bind situation, and that is why they remain silent on the larger issues.

The senior author alone takes responsibility for the following dim view of the dynamics of our society. This miniature diatribe deals with the latent functions of maintaining women in a state of depression, along with minorities, and the importance of having that bottom group of criminals and delinquents to define the limits of our own far from perfect behavior. Every middle class man has his secret Watergate, but a delinquent a day keeps the doctor away. Sporadic unemployment keeps the labor force malleable just as food shortages do worldwide. A 4 percent annual growth rate is no longer possible in the United States, so there must be permanent unemployment (see "Okun's Law," in B. Commoner, 1976). Resistance to day care or family intervention, and the anger over the implied "permissiveness" of psychiatric treatment as opposed to punishment of juveniles or deviants, is laid overtly to invasion of privacy. Covertly, there may be recognition that true changes in family styles might produce upwardly mobile minority children.

The "bottom line" philosphy prevails, but service to people is the first to get the ax. Science has been demoted. Perhaps Mental Health has been upstaged by Drugs and Alcohol, but health *in general* has lost its priority. The national mood, including that of youth, is antiscientific, antipsychological, and antisociological because it is environmental and antitechnological. Science and higher education are tarred with the same brush as technology. The power of the individual is decreasing. His home is now, more than ever, his only castle. Why shouldn't he abuse his wife or children? As in *The Taming of the Shrew*, there's nobody left to kick but the dog. "Revenue sharing," an increasing trend, means less money for health and welfare, more for local roads and buildings, more power locally. These problems are widespread.

It seems that mankind has an insatiable need for power over others, and his means of demonstrating power are growing rapidly. This need may have been first evidenced in human sacrifice as a way of achieving immortality. As Becker (1973) suggests, fear of death may be the motive for the power drive, as expressed in wars and economic exploitation. The excesses of consumption in the face of world starvation, burgeoning overpopulation, vast wars and massive genocide in recent history make our preventive or interventive measures seem pitifully weak.

Can a few trained people offer any help in attacking worldwide social pathology? Should we counsel or promote love, calmness, and consistency in marriage, between friends and among nations, as well as in child-parent relationships? Didn't somebody write something like that before? I seem to recall it dimly.

Geel, Belgium: The Natural Therapeutic Community 1475–1975

Leo Srole

Community psychiatry, as we all know, is a many faceted, incomplete and still pioneering enterprise. At the service level, one of its central commitments is to avoid long term hospitalization of the chronically impaired, accomplished by placing them, whenever necessary, in one of a spectrum of supervised community residential types. The smallest and sociologically most natural of these types is the foster family home, which is also the common ancestor of all other types now gathered under the sheltering umbrella of community psychiatry.

To place the present report in brief historical perspective, we know that foster family care was already in a seedling stage when Europe's first psychiatric hospital, in Valencia, Spain, was established early in the fifteenth century, at the very threshold of the Renaissance. Such family care first emerged on a significant and viable scale in the agricultural crossroads village of Geel in Flanders, not on the professional initiative of a churchman, as in Valencia, nor of a physician as in Pinel's trail blazing hospital in Paris, but of unschooled peasants and burghers in an area of economically marginal land.

These simple folk opened their homes for the transient keep of the mentally ill pilgrims who came for the ritual of the novena at the shrine of Geel's locally canonized St. Dymphna. Local legend has it that Dymphna was the Christian daughter of a pagan Irish king who, upon the death of his Queen, pressed his daughter, seen as the image of her mother, to marry him; whereupon Dymphna fled by boat to the Lowlands. The outraged King, pursuing and catching up with her on the outskirts of Geel, beheaded her for continuing to resist his incestuous suit.

A carved Renaissance panel in the sacristy of Geel's St. Dymphna

Church portrays the deranged King wielding the sword at the prompting of the satanic figure beside him. Thus the daughter came to be seen as paying the price of martyrdom to resist the devil who was possessing and inciting her father. In Geel's earliest extant records, dating from the fifteenth century, mention is already made of pilgrimages of "The Innocents" to the shrine of St. Dymphna. Historians, however, attribute the origin of the legend to the seventh century A.D.

This is not the place to trace the long, subsequent history of Geel's practice of taking the mentally ill into its homes. But several salient details may suggest its evolutionary course:

1. The medieval "possession" theory of mental disorder in Geel, as elsewhere, subsequently evolved into the "sickness" view of behavioral disability.
2. During that evolution, the length of stay of the *ziecke* in Geel homes gradually increased until it sometimes approached permanence.
3. For centuries, the practice of taking the sick into a Geel family was on a boarding basis arranged between the householder and the sick person's kinfolk or other representative—that is, it was informal in nature, although under the loose oversight of the chapter of local canons.
4. In 1836 the practice came under the secular authority and supervision of the Geel Municipal Council, functions assumed in 1850 by the Belgian government, which designated the program formally with the institutional title of Rijkskolonie, or State Colony.
5. In 1862 the Kolonie acquired its first medical framework in the form of a small inpatient facility for initial or interim observation of patients and treatment of their somatic problems. That is, the hospital primarily provided inpatient and ambulatory medical support for patients in foster families, although they were also rehospitalized if the family found them unmanageable.

It is also interesting historically that the first alienist known to visit Geel, in the early 1830s, was Etienne Esquirol, disciple of and successor to Pinel in Paris. Esquirol sharply criticized the Geel program, in part because of the absence of medical care, a condition also shared at the time by the citizens of what was still a village, and in part because he felt that those mentally sick placed in foster families were being deprived of a hospital's unique therapeutic environment and moral treatment regimen.

However, Esquirol was followed after the middle of the nineteenth century by a new breed of alienists, those disillusioned with the mental hospitals in Europe and abroad, who were now in search of practical alternatives to hospitalization. As a result, Geel-like family care programs were established in fourteen European and North American countries, but until recently none replicated Geel's unique ingredient of a "colony," defined by spatial cohesion of foster families in some numbers. Specifically, Geel has a relatively small inpatient facility with numerous patients in the families of a relatively small community.

The town in 1971, the midpoint of our period of data gathering, had a population of approximately 30,000, to which its 1200 family care patients stand in a ratio of about 40 per 1,000 resident population. To put the situation in graphic New York City terms: Manhattan's average four-sided block shelters about 1,000 individuals. Thus, if Geel's patient density rate just mentioned applied there, the average Manhattan block would accommodate about 40 free-living chronic mental patients in its homes and its streets. Here I should also add that the Geel-inspired family care programs elsewhere almost invariably followed a different pattern, revolving around a *large* hospital as hub, but with relatively *few* patients in homes scattered through a *large* area. By contrast, Geel represented cohesion rather than dispersion, high patient-to-population density rather than low density, offering greater opportunity for supervision at lower administrative cost.

Despite the nineteenth century "invasion" of individual alienists who made the professional pilgrimage to Geel, with a continuing impact reflected in the journals of European and American psychiatry for more than a century, none to our knowledge paid more than a quick look-see visit. As a result, the profession heard little more than superficialities and stereotypes about Geel, until American psychiatrists Knight Aldrich and Matthew Dumont spent several weeks in Geel during the summer of 1960. Their visits had three consequences:

1. They published an article in the August 1962 issue of the *American Journal of Psychiatry*, entitled "Family Care After a Thousand Years—A Crisis in the Tradition of St. Dymphna."
2. In 1963 Dr. Jan Schrijvers, a young Belgian psychiatrist and native of Geel, was recruited for training by and in the Columbia Division of Community Psychiatry.
3. In January 1966, under the prompting of my Columbia colleagues, Drs. Lawrence C. Kolb, Viola W. Bernard, and Harry Shapiro, I spent several weeks in Belgium taking soundings on the feasibility

of a study of Geel and its foster family program. I reported back that on the basis of the encouragement I received from top echelons of the Belgian Ministry of Health, the University of Leuven, and the Geel Municipality and Rijkskolonie, such an investigation appeared feasible, but would require a seasoned combination of social anthropologist and psychiatric sociologist to design and direct it. I added that I knew of only one person in all of Belgium and the U.S.A. who qualified with that particular multidisciplinary lineage, and although that person was already fully committed to the Midtown Manhattan Restudy (then in a planning stage), he surely could not resist the unique, untouched, broad scientific attractiveness of Geel.

And so I conflictually trapped myself into the role of the commuting part time Geel Project Director, spending in the next ten years an average of ten weeks annually in that capacity. With this long and unusual background as a prologue, I can now turn to give you a highly selective account of the Geel Project itself and several key findings from our data bank that are pertinent to the theme of this symposium.

Following my January 1966 reconnaisance visit, the Geel research design evolved as a master plan on paper, with Dr. Schrijvers initially as my only local assistant in Geel, with a small budget from the Family Care Foundation for the Mentally Ill and the Foundations Fund for Research in Psychiatry, later supplemented by the support of the New York State Psychiatric Institute, an NIMH International Grant, and allocations from the Belgium Ministry of Health and Leuven University research funds. The scale of the unfolding design appeared beyond practical reach, especially as it would have to hinge entirely on recruiting many competent Flemish-speaking field workers of diverse skills to work part time under the close direction of a commuting scientist from the United States.

In time, the recruited numbered almost 100 people, drawn (1) from the faculty and graduate student ranks of eight departments in the University of Leuven (psychiatry, public health, social psychology, clinical psychology, anthropology, economics, sociology and history), (2) from the Rijkskolonie professional and paraprofessional staffs, (3) from Geel's resident laymen, including eight patients as clerks and concierges in our Project Center, and (4) several Americans from my Columbia staff, all of the above on a fractional time basis.

As an international, interuniversity, interdisciplinary research team operating under restraints of time, money, and personnel availabilities in a country with a population about the size of New York City and Long Island, the Project's forty component study units that we now have completed fill many but by no means all of the facets envisaged in my master plan.

Let me now indicate the Project's overall approach, which was that of a low profile, naturalistic, in vivo study of Geel's foster care patients and major parts of the community milieu that impinge on their day-to-day lives. My overarching question was: how does Geel "do its thing" for its patients, and with what results? However, it was neither scientifically necessary, in my view, nor practicably possible, in the view of my Flemish collaborators, to introduce any quasi-experimental controls into a very old system—especially not by an outside research director, however warmly he was initially received and subsequently accepted in the Geel and Leuven University communities.

Beyond the purely descriptive purpose of portraiture, we had a number of programmatic, policy oriented questions that we wanted answered. Both to Dumond and Aldrich in 1960 and to me in 1966 there appeared to be *extrinsic* factors threatening the long term survival of the Geel program of family care. My second question, therefore, was that of a sociological diagnostician addressing himself to a seemingly ailing institution, namely, what are the pathogenic forces at work, and what counteractive steps should be considered as feedback recommendations to its staff in Geel?

Given the antiquity of the Geel program, and the resistance to change endemic in all deeply rooted institutions, it was almost inevitable that it would lag behind the accelerating pace of psychiatry's research and service developments in the quarter century from 1940 to 1965. My question, therefore, was: what features of recent psychiatric thinking and practice could be integrated into the Geel program without compromising its basic family care principles? I expected, and indeed confirmed, that the Rijkskolonie's errors of omission and commission were correctible, and thereby would be of primary interest to its staff and authorities in the Belgian Ministry of Health.

Third, although foster family care had been on the peripheries of some American mental hospitals since 1888, I posed this more general question in 1966, a year in which funding for America's new community health centers' program was just moving into local pipelines: what sound intrinsics of family care, as exemplified in Geel, can be extended to the American scene in a period of psychiatry's stepped up search for alternatives to hospitalization for chronic mental patients?

Answers to the latter question are emerging from ongoing analysis of data from the forty circumscribed study units that ultimately comprised the mosaic of the less than completely comprehensive Geel Project. These study units fall into the following six main clusters:

1. History of Geel family care and its nurturant community: 1475–1975.
2. Patient composition and changes in the Geel milieu.
3. Foster family structure and process.
4. The Rijkskolonie as an institution: its foster family policies and practices.
5. The Geel community as the embracing extramural surround of the foster family and its patients.
6. Ambivalent images of Geel among Belgian non-Geelians (including mental health professionals), as they impinge on the family care system and on Geel's contrasting images of itself.

In the space remaining to me I can cover only a few highlights from these clusters, namely, (1) a brief description of Geel the community, (2) a short accounting of the characteristics of the patients, (3) the results from one of a series of studies of patient change in Geel, and (4) foster family characteristics and processes.

Let us first get a quick view of Geel, the community. Consulting a national map, we find that it is in the northeast corner of the Flemish-speaking section of Belgium, forty motor car minutes due east of the port of Antwerp and an hour's drive northeast from Brussels. Viewed from a helicopter, the hub of the town is its ancient marketplace, where stand the city hall, the main church, the town's only hotel (vintage 1910), its only cinema, a modern, two-floor department store, and small shops, cafes, and restaurants. Here are held fortnightly open markets, continuing a tradition of a thousand years, as well as periodic carnivals and Sunday band concerts. Shops principally purveying home furnishings, clothing, foodstuffs, and spirits also appear for short distances on several side streets radiating out as spokes from the hub.

Until recently Geel's housing stock was almost entirely single family homes. Immediately circling the marketplace are streets with such houses closely clustered cheek by jowl. Around this tight urban core[a] is a more open belt of suburbanlike dwellings where several 6–7 floor apartment houses have recently intruded. The outermost

[a] In this urban core dwell about half the population.

ring is a broad, green belt, once divided into many small farms, now consolidated into fewer units on larger land holdings.[b]

Scattered through the green belt are establishments for processing and storing products of the land: a slaughterhouse, flour mills, granaries, and the like, survivors of the town's original agrarian economy. At the southwest corner of the green belt, adjoining the super highway to Antwerp, is a large, new, nationally planned and sponsored industrial zone for the high technology factories producing electronics, plastics, frozen foods, that were beginning to rise at my first visit in 1966.

Geel's contemporary occupational structure can be read from the following distribution of its heads of household (HOH) in 1971 (Table 2−7). Note that only about one-fourth of the HOH are in white collar occupations (the top three strata include Rijkskolonie staff in some numbers), almost half are in the blue collar category, and an unexpectedly large one-fourth are out of the labor force but previously had been blue collar workers in the main. The predominant blue collar complexion of this population is certainly clear, a picture reinforced by the fact that 61.5 percent of Geel's HOH had only elementary grade schooling, 21.6 percent had gone to vocational high school, while only 8.2 percent to general high school and 8.7 percent to higher levels of education.

I should emphasize that with the collaboration of several anthropologists and social psychologists, including Professors Leo Lagrou

Table 2−7. Occupational Distribution of Geel's 7700 HOH
(Based on 1971 National Census)

2.4	Professionals, para-professionals
9.0	Manager-administrators
8.0	Other white collar employees
7.0	Self-employed shopkeepers
4.7	Blue collar: farmers
18.8	Blue collar: other technical skills
23.1	Blue collar: unskilled
25.9	Nonemployed: retired, widowed, invalid, etc.
1.1	Unknown
100.0	

Foster parenthood is not classified as an occupation.

Heads of households, rather than total labor force, comprise the universe here, because they were so specified for Geel Project use in the computer tape provided by the Belgian Census agency.

[b]The municipality occupies a total area of about 42 square miles, the largest in Belgium after Brussels and Antwerp; half of it is in the outer green belt.

and Eugene Roosens of the University of Leuven, we have also covered such other sociological dimensions of the Geel community impinging on patients as its twelve parish churches and their affiliated voluntary associations, its public health and mental health aspects, its recreational facilities, and above all, the informal interactions of Geel's citizens and patients in public and semipublic places.

From this overview of the community, I would next turn to a quick scan of the 1200 patients who in 1971 were in Geel's 1060 foster homes. Their age range is from eighteen into the eighties, some having been in local families five decades or more, and number 75 percent males to 25 percent females. Diagnostically about one-third of them are classified on the Rijkskolonie record as chronic functional conditions, principally schizophrenia and the affective disorders, roughly one-third represent organically based retardations, and the rest learning retardations seeming to be secondary to primary personality and/or social pathologies. Most had been hospitalized for varyingly long periods prior to placement in Geel.

Approximately 14 percent are of middle class parentage, several themselves artists or business men, the rest are from blue collar families. In geographic provenience Geel's foster care patients are now largely from other places in Flanders. In previous decades they also included appreciable numbers from the French speaking, southern section of Belgium, and in smaller numbers from other countries as distant as Russia, England, and even the United States.

Having previously observed custodial patients on the wards of traditional American and Belgian hospitals, my first impression of Geel's patients was that (1) they were actively engaged in the business of normal family living, rather than apathetically disengaged, and (2) outer directed in their public behaviors, rather than inaccessibly withdrawn into their private worlds. Clearly no research was necessary to demonstrate that it is more humane and less pathogenic to arrange for such human beings to function spontaneously in a state of freedom, than to wall them up for long stretches of time in a state of numbing captivity, however benign their overseers.

Nevertheless, our main research thrust was to learn how different kinds of patients fare in different kinds of foster families in the open Geel community. To this end, we intensively studied four sets of patients:

1. A prospective followup over 30 months of 64 patients from first placement in a family, using a large battery of tests and relevant interviewing methods. The information is now on computer tape and undergoing complicated statistical analyses.

2. A sample of 48 patients divided evenly between those judged by informed staff to have improved most, and those who had done most poorly since their placement two or more years earlier. They were tested once in a cross-sectional design that focused on isolating the factors that could account for the previous differential changes of the two subsamples.
3. A sample of 64 patients transferred from the Kortenberg Hospital, one of the best in Belgium, to Geel families, with followup assessment in a range from six months to seven years later.
4. Twenty-four ex-patients discharged to their home communities, interviewed and tested a year or more after discharge to learn how they were functioning in their native environment.

Three of the above study units were conducted by Miss Godlieve Vercruysse, of the University of Leuven, and Dr. Jan Schrijvers. Here I can report only about the Kortenberg study unit, which has been presented in a paper by Professor Roland Pierloot,[c] Chairman of the University of Leuven Department of Psychiatry, Director of the Kortenberg Hospital, and, along with Professors Jan Blanpain and Joseph Nuttin, one of the Project's three Belgian Advisors from 1966 onward.[d]

The average length of hospitalization among the 64 Kortenberg transferees to Geel had been ten years. Primarily excluded from transfer were patients considered generally unsuited for family life, e.g., marked by "disturbing or dangerous behavior, such as regular aggressive outbursts, sexual acting-out, suicide attempts or addictions, [and lacking] a sufficient autonomy in elementary functions (eating, dressing, toilet) and a minimum of stable integration into some form of occupational therapy in the hospital." Even so, Dr. Pierloot notes, "in the large majority of these patients the prospects of clinical improvement were considered as very limited." He further describes them as "predominantly female, mostly middle-aged, stabilized [chronic] schizophrenics and personality disorders on the basis of mental retardation, for whom returning to their natural milieu seemed excluded." Outcomes at final followup, classified by Dr. Pierloot on information gathered by "the doctors and sector nurses in Geel," were as shown in Table 2–8.

All in all, only the five rehospitalized for reasons other than lan-

[c]R.A. Pierloot and M. Demarsin, "Significance of Geel Foster Family Care to Patients of a Psychiatric Hospital," paper presented to International Symposium on Foster Family Care, Geel, Belgium, May 16, 1975.

[d]The Project's American Advisors have been Professors Viola W. Bernard, Lawrence C. Kolb and Harry Shapiro, all of Columbia University.

Table 2—8.   Outcomes at Followup of 64 Kortenberg Patient Transferees to Geel Foster Families

2	Died
4	Returned to Kortenberg Hospital after short trial stay in Geel family (primarily because they were French speaking and had difficulties with Flemish
5	Rehospitalized elsewhere
4	Returned to natural family
49	"Relatively well integrated" in a Geel foster family, with symptoms of—

      6 no longer manifest
    14 at "moderate" level
    29 at "serious" level

guage difficulties can be regarded as "failures" of the foster family to prevent rehospitalization. Moreover, of the 49 patients remaining in Geel, Dr. Pierloot comments that "the social functioning of 80 to 85 percent can be considered as enriched and more differentiated." As for preference between foster family and hospital care, these patients chose as follows (Table 2—9):

Important is the professionally observed quality of the interaction between patient and foster mother, as revealed in the following distribution (Table 2—10). Two further facts should be added: (1) with few exceptions, all of these patients were continued by the Kortenberg Hospital staff on more or less the same drug regimen as before transfer; and (2) there is generally little direct psychiatric input from

Table 2—9.   Remaining Patients' Preferred Place of Care

29	Foster family
5	Hospital
<u>15</u>	Either
49	

Table 2—10.   Remaining Patients' Quality of Interaction with Geel Foster Mother

35	Positive
9	Neutral
<u>5</u>	Negative (same patients as "preferred hospital")
49	

the Rijkskolonie physicians to the Geel patient or his foster family. Thus, we can conclude that such symptomatic, social functioning and attitudinal changes as came about in these 49 patients can probably be largely attributed to the array of characteristics differentiating the hospital and Geel's foster family milieus.

Also relevant is that these changes occurred despite the fact that we have discerned considerable room for improvement in the Rijkskolonie's procedures (1) of screening applicant families into its program, (2) of matching patient characteristics to the therapeutically most appropriate kind of family, (3) of helping to bridge the initial "stranger distance" between the newly placed patient and his foster family, and (4) of enlarging foster parent insights into, and goal setting for, the patient. In the light of these four correctible program deficiencies, the changes observed in the 49 Kortenberg transferees are all the more a noteworthy achievement of the Geel foster family, as it operates almost entirely on its own spontaneous devices, guided by uncodified local experience.

These conclusions lead me to the fourth cluster of Project study units, namely those focused squarely on foster family structure and processes. Even superficial observation indicates the following main facts about the place made for the patient in the foster home:

1. He occupies a bedroom of his own that is an integral part of the dwelling, yet facilitates privacy at will.
2. He shares the family table at mealtime and much of its intramural leisure time activity, including that of watching TV together.
3. He participates, although not as much today as previously, in the family's domestic and income yielding work, thereby supplementing the relatively modest direct payments to the foster family made by the state or other agencies.

To penetrate beyond these surface apparencies, we mounted six different study units to encompass as many different dimensions of the foster family. The first of these dimensions was assigned to Dr. Ferdinand Cuvelier, a social psychologist and specialist in group dynamics. It was his task to observe and audio-tape a sample of 32 foster families and their intrafamily interactions during a sample of days over a span of eight to twelve months after a new patient had been placed in the home. His primary objective was to identify the patterns of behavior by which a disabled stranger is gradually converted into and incorporated as an integral, functional member of the family. This is an outcome that other data indicate has occurred in about half of all foster families.

Let me summarize Dr. Cuvelier's report[e] in terms of a number of generalizations about the newly placed patient in such a family:

1. Feeling rejected by his natural family, community and previous hospital keepers, the patient arrives as, in effect, a rootless drifter and homeless orphan.
2. He experiences the foster family as a normal home, devoid (except in a two-patient home) of other patients, doctors, or even any kind of apparent psychotherapeutic strategy on the part of the foster parents.
3. The latter accept him into their round of daily activities and appropriately correct and reward his behavior in a natural context where he can be himself.
4. The patient is motivated to project himself as someone who behaves well, thereby making himself valued, a value he needs desperately for his severely damaged self-esteem.
5. He gradually takes on the role of a family member—the most basic process being the interpersonal accommodation which calls for considerate, informal give-and-take flexibility on both sides. This two-way flexibility and mutual support often leads to a strong affective bond that undeniably is the most important feature of optimal family care.
6. As the patient identifies with the group ego and collective self his own identity is developed and strengthened. He thereby rejects himself less and invests more energy in his own self.
7. By acquiring ego strength the patient learns to model and adapt himself to the demands reality imposes, helped by the constant influence of the foster family. From this he learns how he can fulfill new roles.
8. The principles involved closely resemble present day behavioral therapy, which in the Geel context can be called more generally "family member therapy."

As a social anthropologist I had long held that the natural, healthy family is psychologically the most counter-pathic institution devised by man. From my first visit onward this seemed preeminently the case in many Geel foster families I had observed. Here I saw not the medical model of the psychiatrist in the fireman's relatively intensive but episodic role of controlling an emotional conflagration; rather, what I did see was a combination of the low keyed, continuing role

[e]F. Cuvelier, "Patterns of Interaction Between Mental Patient and Caretakers," paper presented to International Symposium on Foster Family Care, Geel, Belgium, May 16, 1975.

of the teacher who patiently instructs and guides a slow pupil, and the even more sustained imprinting role of emotionally supportive, reality-knowledgeable behavioral models.

To test those impressions independently of Dr. Cuvelier's study I wanted the clinical judgment of an outside psychiatrist. For this purpose I called in Dr. Jozef Hes, a Dutch reared Israeli psychiatrist who had been trained in social psychiatry under Dr. Fritz Redlich at Yale. Since Dr. Hes has a thorough command of the local language, I turned him loose on his own for several weeks to visit Geel foster families, at random and unannounced, for freewheeling interviews and observations of how family and patient relate to each other.

Like other Project investigators, Dr. Hes was surprised that some families in the program had ever been accepted for patient care. On the other hand, he also found Geel care givers who are exemplars of the normalizing, socializing, destigmatizing, parent-teacher role that is crucial to raise ego-damaged, behaviorally disabled patients to higher levels of social functioning. In Dr. Hes' opinion, and mine, these care givers represent parenthood at its universal best under the trying circumstances of having a handicapped dependent to bring up normally. Accordingly, they offer a model to the Rijkskolonie and other family care programs elsewhere to extend this standard, and to undergird it with insight training into patient differences and the foster parent's own larger rehabilitating potentialities.

At this point, let us next examine the foster families as a group within the large context of Geel's total of 7700 family units. For this purpose we had the important help of the Belgian National Census of 1971. To the enumeration sheet of that census we arranged to add twenty questions of our own that were asked at all Geel households. This special information, plus the regular demographic data of the census on the same households, the Belgian government has generously made available to us in computer tape format. To this tape we have added information gathered from Rijkskolonie records[f] that permit us to classify all Geel households on the foster family status typology indicated in Table 2–11.

Thus, 15 percent of all Geel families were either in or intended entering the local patient care system, and another 6 percent had retired from it, largely because of advancing age of the parents. Parenthetically, prior to World War II the corresponding frequency of CFF in the community was close to 25 percent. Next, we might

[f]We acknowledge our indebtedness to Mr. Georges Hedebouw, University of Leuven, for his patient and skilled services in interdigitating three sets of information into a single data matrix, and for directing computer output of cross-tabulations on the foster family typology and differentiating characteristics.

focus entirely on the CFF aggregate and ask this question: from what demographic sources in the community have CFF member units primarily been self-recruited? For this purpose I shall draw on data that are being analyzed by my Columbia colleague, Mrs. Anita Fischer.[g]

In several of the following small tables we classify families by the demographic characteristics of the head of household (HOH). To facilitate comparisons we standardize differential frequency rates of CFF by taking the raw percentage of CFF in each population subgroup as numerator and dividing it by the 13.5 percent in Table 2–11 taken as the denominator. This converts the latter percentage into a standard value of 100. To illustrate, raw CFF percentages of 6.75 and 27 percent would be converted into standardized CFF frequency rates of 50 and 200 respectively.

We see that the rates increase with HOH age, ages 45 and 55 appearing as major frequency turning points. However, if frequencies below the 45-year line are by no means negligible, they are certainly open to enlargement by Rijkskolonie recruitment efforts not yet

Table 2–11.   Distribution of Geel's 7700 Households on a Four-fold Typology of Foster Family Status *(Year 1971)*

13.5%	Current Foster Families (CFF)
5.5[a]	Ex-Foster Families
1.6	Applied-to-be Foster Families
79.4	All Other Families
100.0%	

[a]Under the impetus of computerization, the Rijkskolonie's record keeping has vastly improved since 1970. The register of ex-foster families before that is held to be incomplete and this count is accordingly an understatement. The count of All Other Families is therefore correspondingly overstated.

Table 2–12.   CFF Standardized Frequency Rates, by Age of Head of Household (HOH)

Under 35	20
35–44	78
45–54	125
55–64	153
Over 64	162

[g]A.K. Fischer and R. Biel, "Geel Family Typology: Some Characteristics and Attitudes of Foster Families," paper presented to International Symposium on Foster Family Care, Geel, Belgium, May 16, 1975.

attempted. This age picture is elaborated when we look at the corresponding rates by marital status (Table 2—13).

The rate among the widowed reflects two different tendencies: (1) the tendency of a foster parent to continue keeping the patient after his/her spouse has died, and (2) the tendency of nonfostering widows to take a patient for reasons of both companionship and supplementation of reduced income. These motives can be subsumed under the concept of a need to make a "broken home" whole. The same notion can be restated as the need to complete an incomplete family among the unmarrieds, who appear at first glance with a frequency rate higher than might have been anticipated.

The motive of making an incomplete or broken home whole is also seen in the following CFF frequencies, where families are classified by number of occupants (other than patients) in the household (Table 2—14). The peak rate in two-member households primarily reflects "empty nest" or childless couples, or the widowed with a child remaining in the home. For childless couples in particular, a patient offers the opportunity to acquire the otherwise unavailable parent role indispensible to a complete family.

I have referred to supplementation of income as a motive for taking a patient. One facet of this motive in a community of predominantly limited incomes is the family goal of buying a home otherwise not at all possible from its regular source of income, or a home larger than otherwise possible. We know that roughly 70 percent of Geel's "All Other Families" (Table 2—11) own their own home. We lack a corresponding national figure, but I have been given

Table 2—13. CFF Standardized Frequency Rates, by Marital Status of HOH

Unmarried	80
Married	100
Widowed	113

Table 2—14. CFF Standardized Frequency Rates, by Occupants in Household

1	98
2	117
3	85
4	78
5+	114

impressionistic information that this more or less approximates the total home ownership rate of surrounding towns in Geel's arrondissement. Assuming this impression is more or less correct, it is noteworthy that the home ownership rate in Geel's CFF group is 91.5 percent—i.e., almost universal.

Parenthetically, it is commonplace for a Geel foster family to tell visitors that "our patient paid for this house" or "he put our son through university." Actually, the per diem rates paid the foster family for keeping each patient have been relatively modest, and were accrued and forwarded at quarterly intervals. This encouraged the family to bank the payments in its savings account, where in time they accumulated in sufficient amount to provide the margin needed to buy a desired house or pay a child's college tuition.

Having previously noted the occupational distribution of Geel's totality of 7,700 heads of household (Table 2−7), it may be instructive to examine the standardized CFF rates in each occupational category separately (Table 2−15). All occupational strata without exception are represented with foster families, but peak rates emerge in the two strata where income supplementation is an especially strong impetus, namely farmers and the nonemployed. Among farmers, moreover, a related consideration is that a male patient can help to increase productivity or to replace a son moving out to college or a higher occupational career.

Current economic motives for foster parenthood are clearly important, but are in no way diminished by the fact that family tradition also plays a part. By way of explanation, we conducted interviews with heads of household in a 50 percent sample of all CFF. From one series of questions the following frequencies of kin of the CFF couple were reported as ever having been foster parents.

In these frequencies, we directly discern the continuity of the

Table 2−15. CFF Standardized Frequency Rates,
by Occupation of HOH

0.4	Professionals
29.0	Manager-administrators
44.0	Other white collar employees
75.0	Self-employed shopkeepers
450.0	Blue collar: farmers
56.0	Blue collar: other technical skills
87.0	Blue collar: unskilled
142.0	Nonemployed

foster care tradition down four lineal generations, and across two degrees of collateral kinship—i.e., own siblings and parents' siblings. Through our interviews we have for the first time pieced together these four recent generations[h] as visible bearers of a tradition of patient care giving in the processional of Geel families preceding them in unbroken ranks stretching back to the fifteenth century. Stated in most simple contemporary terms, growing up with a patient in one's parents' house, and/or in the home(s) of close kin, tends to prompt, rather than deter, an adult to also carry foster parenthood into his/her own home. Such promptings were an additional factor among CFF in volunteering to assume that role.

However, a significant number of approximately 25 percent of all CFF had no such kinship tradition at all. Are the latter perhaps native born Geelians mainly, who were exposed from early childhood to numerous mental patients in neighboring and other local homes, thereby conditioning them to favor the foster parent role for themselves? To answer this question, we return to the 1971 census data where we can divide all household heads into Geel born and immigrants from elsewhere in Flanders. The latter frequency is based on the absolute number of 271 foster parent couples who were *not* regularly exposed to mental patients at large until they arrived in Geel,

Table 2–16. Percentages of CFF Kin Who Had Ever Been Foster Parents

Percent	
65	with grandparents on either or both sides of the current foster family couple
72	with parents of either or both members of the CFF couple
75	with one or more aunts and/or uncles of either or both members of the CFF couple
65	with one or more siblings of either or both members of the CFF couple
62	with one or more married children of the CFF couple living in Geel

Table 2–17. CFF Standardized Frequency Rates, by HOH Place of Birth

Geel	130
Elsewhere	62

[h] Interestingly, if Geelians have themselves perceived the extent of this kinship chain, none of them, not even those who were my close research collaborators, has given the slightest sign of awareness of its existence.

usually as adults. This evidence bears witness that neither a family tradition, nor nativity in Geel sans such a tradition, is necessary to seek, acquire and hold the foster parent role.

As already reported above, economic considerations are embedded in the tangle of motivations leading Geel born people into patient care careers, and we infer that such considerations are also operating among CFF couples new to Geel. Completion of an incomplete nuclear family structure, and availability of direct and indirect remunerative rewards not otherwise available for such an intrafamily function, probably are the most general motivations cutting across all segments of the CFF population of parents.

I emphasize this point because many outsiders advance the argument that Geel's five-century tradition is historically unique and therefore the program cannot be replicated in or adapted to other places. If that high patient density, communitywide program is viewed as a continuously renewed local experiment as to the possible in human behavior, Geel itself demonstrates the success of the experiment and its intrinsic replicability elsewhere.

The Project's own data add support to the inference that Geel-type programs for chronic mental patients are generalizable to other communities that either lack such a tradition, or are, like Geel today, heterogenous in socioeconomic composition. Furthermore, from the fact that five of every six CFF heads of household had not gone beyond elementary school we can also conclude that the capacity for successful foster parenthood, as indeed for natural parenthood, is largely independent of years of education. In a sense, therefore, Geel long ago anticipated the recent American movement to engage indigenous people of limited education to serve as paraprofessional aides in community mental health programs.

In my opinion, the Geel experience conveys several broad policy implications to the rest of the psychiatric and concerned lay worlds:

1. A foster family program with an ultimate patient density of 40 per thousand resident population is feasible, if instituted slowly and with thorough community preparation and participation.
2. The greater the patient density, (a) the closer and more cost-efficient can be the professional and paraprofessional services for families and patients in the system, (b) the greater can be the secondary identification with or involvement of non-foster families in the system, and (c) the larger can be the sharing of other local institutions in furthering the goals of the system.
3. Inclusive community populations can be socialized from childhood on, primarily by adult example, to behave humanely, with-

out a reflexive, rejecting sense of threat or fear in the presence of emotionally impaired but socially functioning mental patients in some numbers.

4. Under the three conditions just outlined, an entire heterogenous population, even one largely urbanized (as Geel now is), can spontaneously function as a *natural therapeutic community* for those heretofore terminally consigned to hospital wards.

5. Such a community program may also serve functions of a reparative nature for its indigenous families who suffer deficits of resources for their own needs and aspirations.

Having outlined general policy implications for the psychiatric world, I will close by noting three other outputs of the Geel Project:

1. Specifically pinpointed policy recommendations to the Rijkskolonie staff and its Brussels superiors have been made (some already implemented) and others will follow.

2. Monographs by my collaborators are in preparation for professional audiences, each of which will report one of the Project's series of six clusters of study units identified earlier. The Project's Omnibus volume will synthesize the findings of all six of these clusters, in a semipopular, illustrated format targeted to both the lay and professional communities. Its title will be *Community Remarkable of the Western World: Geel, Belgium, 1475–1975.*

3. This chapter in the *Proceedings* of the Kittay 1976 Symposium is the Project's publication debut before an international audience.

Discussant: Social Epidemiology and the Evaluation of Clinical Services

Elmer L. Struening

This discussion is concerned with the implications of the papers presented by Drs. Dohrenwend, Langner, and Srole for what I believe to be some of the goals of community mental health, including the understanding of factors involved in the delivery of services to catchment area populations. My first section will be reactions to the three papers; the second section will focus on a method for understanding relationships between the results of field epidemiological studies and the selective use of clinical services, as the service delivery system is systematically varied.

DOHRENWEND

Dr. Dohrenwend's review and critique of true prevalence studies suggests that the yield from such studies, in terms of the consistency of rates estimates and the magnitude of their relationships with social, cultural, and individual attributes, is indeed meager. The extent to which one can make generalizations about social class, sex, and rural-urban effects, especially in the absence of valid estimates of their magnitudes, would seem to be insufficient justification for conducting expensive field epidemiological studies of mental disorders.

Certainly, there does not appear to be a steady accumulation of knowledge, acceptable to the scientific community, about the distribution and correlates of mental disorders in defined populations. Why is this so? Dr. Dohrenwend raised the crucial issue of the enormous variability among epidemiology investigators in their conceptualization and measurement of mental disorders. Such variation, of course, severely limits the comparability of study results and the pos-

The author thanks Dr. Judith G. Rabkin for her considerable contribution to this paper and Mrs. Mattie L. Jones for preparing the manuscript.

sibility of generalizations so important to the development of a firm knowledge base.

I believe this state of affairs is no longer necessary. Enough is now known about the measurement of psychiatric symptomology to select a set of measures acceptable to a majority of investigators. A comprehensive and critical review of this literature by specialists in applied psychometric procedures and in the measurement of psychiatric symptoms would provide a basis for the selection of items that systematically sample the domain of symptoms, and which meet high standards of interjudge reliability at the item level, in addition to appropriate standards of internal consistency at the scale level.

Special attention should be given to the problem of measuring rare or infrequent but highly important symptoms in a general population, so that subjects selected from a community population are accurately and meaningfully differentiated. The stability of symptoms over different periods of time should be established to identify relatively more transient and more stable symptom patterns. Explicit standards for collecting information form resident populations, with special attention given to effects due to variation in cultural (ethnic, religious) and individual (sex, age) variables, would be needed to insure the development of comparable data sets.

While other considerations could be listed, the important issue is the development of measures of high quality, designed to differentiate resident populations, and acceptable to a majority of investigators. A common core of knowledge derived from each study and collected with standardized instruments would generate the necessary comparable data sets for making more general conclusions. If epidemiological field studies are to have more influence on our understanding of the distribution of untreated mental disorders, their findings must meet the standards of the scientific community and the critical layman.

Community psychiatry emphasizes the need to understand the communities we serve, especially the variation in mental health status over different sectors of societies. As Dr. Dohrenwend's paper indicates, our current level of knowledge is inadequate. Cooperation among leaders in psychiatric epidemiology and psychometric methods, together with the enlightened support of the National Institute of Mental Health, are needed to develop this important field.

Dr. Dohrenwend is concerned with both the concurrent and sequential relationships of physical and mental illness. While I share his interest, I believe the problem should be conceptualized in a larger framework, with implications for the validity of epidemiological studies. Social stress theory and empirical studies, particularly as formulated and synthesized by Selye (1976) and Cassel (1975), provide considerable evidence for the general hypothesis that stressful conditions produce nonspecific outcomes. That is, members of a population may react to stress environmental conditions by manifesting a variety of physical and mental symptoms, sequentially or in combination, or by displaying patterns of deviant behavior. Cassel and Leighton (1969) note appropriately that it may be necessary in field epidemiological studies to measure a complete range of potential reactions to social stress.

If only a limited range of potential reactions to social stressors are observed, then important types of reaction may be missed and inferences regarding the possible effects of community conditions and family and social structure may be misleading. As both Cobb (1974) and Mechanic (1974) have concluded, both from their studies and those of others, physical and mental symptoms are intimately related, occurring together and sequentially. To observe one domain and not the other may lead us to erroneous conclusions when, in fact, individuals of different background simply express their reactions to stressors in different terms (Thomas and Garrison, 1975). While it seems necessary to study the whole person in terms of a range of meaningful reactions to social stressors, it is not comforting to think that field epidemiology studies must become even more complex in both scope and content.

Epidemiological field studies have traditionally accepted symptom manifestation and, more recently, role performance, as dependent or outcome variables. Sociodemographic variables, including ethnicity, social class, migration, rural-urban residence, sex, age, and marital status, have been conceptualized as independent or classification variables for purposes of comparison or correlation. The development of life events and social stress research has influenced us to conceptualize and measure aspects of the environment thought to be related to the onset of physical or mental illness.

It has been demonstrated to the satisfaction of many investigators that extreme conditions of biological and psychological duress, such as those experienced by concentration camp inmates or Japanese POWs during World War II, cause both physiological and psychiatric disabilities of a generally chronic nature in virtually all who were exposed. Thus, social-environmental conditions apparently *can* cause illness in the absence of other factors commonly presumed to be necessary in disease onset.

However, under ordinary conditions of living it is becoming increasingly apparent that physical and mental illness susceptibility is the product of multiple conditions and their interactions, including:

1. Not simply the occurrence but the *clustering* of life events in a relatively short span of time.
2. The presence of inadequate or deficient social support systems that ordinarily serve as buffers or protectors against stressful life events.
3. The occurrence of *extreme* or *prolonged* stressful life events.
4. Deficient personal resources or lack of prior experience and preparation for the stressful life event(s).
5. Low biological and psychological thresholds.
6. In the case of an infectious disease, the presence of a disease agent.

In short, knowledge of the nature of life events experienced by a defined population is insufficient to accurately identify individuals who will respond with physical or psychiatric disorders.

It seems necessary to understand the interactions of individual attributes with an ever changing social and environmental context if we are to predict important and significant proportions of variability in outcome, such as illness onset. While I would like to share more of Dr. Dohrenwend's enthusiasm for life events research, I find it difficult to be optimistic after a critical review of current research. The review by Rabkin and Struening, (in press) including the excellent critiques of Drs. Bruce and Barbara Dohrenwend, indicates that on the average, less than 10 percent of the variation in illness onset is explained from a knowledge of life event measures.

If social conditions other than life events were appropriately controlled, it is doubtful if many of the life events–illness onset relationships would reach significance. Thus for life events research to mature into a predictive science it must consider more of the complexity of the social context in which the events occur, particularly the nature of support systems.

LANGNER

The work of Dr. Langner and his colleagues represents significant advances in field epidemiological studies. Among the issues I would like to discuss are those concerning Dr. Langner's use of empirically determined profiles as a method for behavioral description in contrast to the use of traditional diagnostic categories, the reliability and validity of this approach, and the question of optimal use of available treatment resources, once children with problems are identified by means of behavioral profiles.

Dr. Langner's research incorporates the following achievements:

1. Identification of 18 reliable and relatively independent dimensions of child behavior, by factor analysis, of over 200 observations gathered from parent interviews.
2. Organization of scores on these 18 dimensions into profiles that describe patterns of behavioral disorders in children. Once standardized, scores on these profiles were used to compare individuals and identify those with similar profiles as behavior types.
3. By using a prospective longitudinal design, Dr. Langner was able to identify relatively transient behavioral disturbances as well as more enduring patterns. That is, he was able to determine what variables on an earlier occasion were effective predictors of later behavior, and which variables on the earlier occasion signified short-lived behavior patterns.

Dr. Langner's eschewal of traditional diagnostic categories in favor of empirically determined dimensions of behavior raises the old controversy regarding the relative reliability, validity, and utility of these two strategies of behavioral description. I believe that his present work demonstrates the strengths of the former methods in each of these respects.

For research purposes, where the problems of reliability and validity necessarily haunt the researcher, the direct route from ratings or observations to their empirical organization into dimensions and summary scores seems to be less hazardous and less subject to a number of sources of error.

Diagnosis represents an attempt to classify a selected sample of observations and inferences into a diagnostic category usually defined as a related cluster of symptoms or behaviors. In the process of making a diagnosis, or categorical judgement, each diagnostician not only elicits and observes a different sample of behavior but also organizes and weighs this sample of observations and inferences according to a highly individualized set of assumptions. In addition there lurk in the shadows the inevitable effects due to differences between the interviewer and subject in sex, social class, ethnicity, age, cultural values, social desirability of symptoms, and others.

It should be self-evident as to why there is little agreement among mental health professionals (Spitzer, 1975) in their assignment of diagnostic labels, except under conditions where they are extensively trained within a very specific diagnostic system, including at least partially structured interviews and detailed instructions for making conclusions.

In contrast, Dr. Langner's system of classifications is straightforward. It asks a large number of very specific questions about a sample of behavior assumed to be relevant and important to the child's adjustment, both concurrently and with implications for the future. The organization of respondents' replies to interview questions is empirically determined. While some personal judgement is required in making data analytic decisions, such as the question of how many factors to rotate, the total process is essentially objective and easily replicated on other samples to assess the generality of results. Samples of behavior organized into a cluster may then be scored and summed into a total score which then distributes the sample of subjects on a continuum of deviant behavior.

The internal consistency reliability of each dimension is easily computed, as illustrated in Dr. Langner's presentation, providing the investigator with important information on the limitations of each measure of behavior. Standardized profiles of behavior can be compared and analyzed with multivariate clustering methods to yield *types* of behavior patterns. The types identified in a population are analogous to diagnostic categories, with the distinct advantage of being based on a series of measures with known reliability. In Dr. Langner's study we recall that the identified types are based on a profile of 18 dimensions of observation.

All this work is of little value unless the identified and measured dimensions and types are valid and useful in the understanding and predicting of behavior. Dr. Langner approached the problem of face and content validity by a detailed review of what other investigators believed were aspects of behavior important to the adjustment of children. The identification of 18 meaningful and reliable dimensions of behavior supports high standards of content validity, although, of course, there may be other important dimensions of behavior which were not identified and which may emerge in subsequent work.

The demonstration of concurrent validity (Gersten et al., 1976), based on the multiple correlation of the 18 dimensions with psychiatric ratings of impairment derived from a review of the mother's report, would appear highly satisfactory. The level of agreement between psychiatric ratings based on direct examination and ratings based on a review of the mother's report is disturbingly low. Obviously, these two procedures provide very different samples of information for the rater.

Probably the most important characteristics of a set of measures are their predictive and construct validity. Dr. Langner's report indicates high standards of long term prediction, especially when the possible effects of maturation on the predictability of children's behavior is considered. I suspect that studies in progress, involving the testing of more specific hypotheses, will continue to substantiate the construct validity of the various sets of measures developed in the work of Dr. Langner and colleagues.

In summary, Dr. Langner has demonstrated how reliable, valid, and theoretically meaningful measures of behavioral disorders of children can be developed by using highly respected multivariate methods which, as he notes, have been in the literature for over 20 years. The resulting measures represent a complex conception of childrens' deviant behavior which would indeed be difficult to force into a categorical labeling system. It is time for ancient and unworkable categorical systems to yield to more scientific and useful classification systems that, to a greater extent, approximate the complexity of children's behavior and avoid the stereotypes of narrowly defined diagnostic labels.

Dr. Langner's work demands replication in different populations to establish the generality of the psychometric properties of his measures. As previously indicated, standardized measures with psychometric properties acceptable to the scientific community are necessary to place field epidemiological studies on a firmer foundation that allows the comparison of study results, the accurate estimation of population parameters, and the development of predictive studies.

As a postscript to Dr. Langner's research, it is important to note that he raises an issue which, though not new, is both dramatic and disturbing. In his sample, he and his colleagues found that only half of the severely impaired children were ever referred to any type of service, and only 20 percent of those referred were seen more than once or twice. These children were not seen as needing help by their schools, their parents, or any other group who came into contact with them.

What is also troubling is the realization that existing facilities for child treatment in New York City are already overburdened, and nothing is "left over" for these unidentified and untreated children in terms of resources. As Ryan (1969) observed with respect to comparable findings in a Boston survey, "there is no place, there are no people, there is no time available to them" (p. 12). In short, as Langner notes, we don't have the personnel and money to take care of those children who are already identified as impaired. How, then, can we finance new programs?

If we devote our attention and services to primary prevention programs, even assuming that we know how to "prevent" the development of disorders in children and families that might otherwise cost more to treat in the future in the absence of intervention programs, what is to become of the "generation" of people who are already impaired? This is a major strategic and moral problem that faces not only practitioners of community psychiatry, but also those in medicine, education, and all programs addressed to the amelioration of social disorders.

SROLE

Dr. Srole's paper raises a set of crucial issues in the development of community psychiatry programs. Foremost among them is the development of community settings for former mental patients. Faced with the general failure of the mental hospital system as it is currently conceptualized, financed, administered, and monitored, mental health administrators are being forced, through court decree or financial necessity, to develop new community structures in which former, usually long term mental patients can achieve a respectable level of adjustment. How can this best be done?

In describing a series of studies aimed at understanding and evaluating the Geel Therapeutic Community (GTC), Dr. Srole has identified conditions and procedures that might enhance the probability of a successful therapeutic community based on a foster home care concept. For example, Dr. Srole suggests that the economic marginality of Geel played an important role in the acceptance of the mentally disabled. That is, some mixture of altruism and pragmatism were key issues in the success of the GTC.

This raises a more general question: in other settings, are economically marginal families who need to augment their marginal incomes a desirable population from which to select and train foster families? While Dr. Srole's research cannot be expected to answer this more general question, it seems likely that his evaluation of the effectiveness of foster homes, within the GTC, will result in evaluation methods which can be applied in other settings.

Another issue raised by Dr. Srole's paper is that of preferred patient density in community settings. Should we create community settings with a relatively large proportion of former patients, such as the GTC, or should former patients be integrated into the community in relatively small numbers? Theoretical advantages and disadvantages could be developed for both positions. Unfortunately, with the pressure to place so many former patients in communities, both points of view are being acted on, with little attention given to their relative effectiveness or the rationale, assumptions, and value systems that they represent.

Especially refreshing is Dr. Srole's spelling out of the structural conditions assumed important to a successful foster care program.

Somehow the humanistic and structural requirements necessary to the effective rehabilitation of mental patients are conspicuously absent in many of our treatment settings. The concern of community psychiatry with continuity of care represents one attempt to help patients experience a sequence of therapeutic events which facilitates their reintegration into their original communities or, if this fails, into a new community setting, as illustrated by the GTC.

Dr. Srole's paper raises an even more general issue. How do we identify and effectively use the many support systems that do exist in different kinds of communities? This is obviously a concern of community psychiatry—a concern of considerable complexity, but one nevertheless that is being faced, however reluctantly, by mental health professionals.

While the mental health establishment can provide some measure of help to people with psychiatric problems, it can never hope to adequately serve those with even severe mental disorders, as indicated by the work of Langner and Ryan (1969). Therefore we need to identify those positive forces in communities which can lower the incidence of psychiatric disorders as well as help and accept those unfortunate enough to experience them. While providing psychological bandaids, we need to learn more about social resources which prevent and ameliorate mental disorders. If mental health professionals do not provide leadership in such attempts, who will?

Dr. Srole's paper describes a specific instance of the historical development of a therapeutic community in a particular village in a particular nation. The *N* is *ONE*. Whether or not we can generalize from his results to communities in other countries remains to be seen. Considering the remarkable history and accomplishments of the citizens of Geel, a full documentation of this history and identification of the reasons for its success and survival seems to me a very worthy goal in itself.

Perhaps we can look forward to a general methodology for evaluating the effectiveness of foster home programs, complete with the identification of former patient and home characteristics which result in maximum and minimum levels of rehabilitation, plus an understanding of the relationships of the program members to the social structure and value system of the larger community, including its social and mental health support systems. Perhaps we could also give up the artificial debate between community psychiatry and "other psychiatry" and focus our attention on the effectiveness of mental health programs which, presumably, do serve people living in communities, whatever their structure and location.

In other words, we are stuck with the reality that people live in communities which influence their lives profoundly, in both a negative and positive manner. We are currently engaged in a movement of long term patients into communities and in a policy of brief hospitalization not because of humanistic values but because long term hospitalization has become too expensive, doesn't work, and is probably necessary for only a small percentage of patients. This rapid movement of former patients into communities is being done with little attention to the results of evaluation studies in this area.

This places community programs in jeopardy because of the lack of informed planning and subsequent evaluation. We face the possibility of the haphazard development of community residential programs, without adequate evaluation and accountability, leading once again, as in the case of mental hospitals, to adverse community reaction, legal intervention, court directives, and a cynical public which is being asked to foot a large mental health budget. Do we ever learn?

EPIDEMIOLOGY AND THE DELIVERY OF CLINICAL SERVICES

One purpose of field epidemiological studies of true prevalence is to identify people in community populations with mental disorders who presumably need some form of clinical treatment. One purpose of clinical services is to provide a form of treatment to members of a population, frequently the residents of a catchment area, who are experiencing mental disorders.

What is the relationship between identification of disorders by field epidemiologists and self/other selection for referral and treatment by community members? What should this relationship be? Should clinical services be designed to seek out the high risk groups identified by field epidemiologists? What types of clinical service delivery systems will most effectively meet the needs of high risk groups as determined by epidemiological surveys?

These questions address themselves to the relationship between true and treated prevalence rates and how the latter would be affected by innovations and changes in the delivery of clinical services. Their answers would seem to be the joint, cooperative responsibility of community mental health administrators and clinicians, social epidemiologists, and program evaluators.

In what follows I shall outline a set of procedures for understanding the selective use of clinical services by catchment area members, and for identifying patterns of clinical service use as they relate to the results of field epidemiological studies.

Description of the Catchment Area:
Independent Variables

One approach to the understanding of relationships between community characteristics and the selective use of clinical services is that of social area analysis (Struening, 1975; Brandon, 1975). It may be viewed as a form of social epidemiology because of the focus on relationships among socioenvironmental characteristics of defined social areas, and the health and mental health status of social area residents.

Assume that our hypothetical clinical service system is serving a catchment area of 400,000 residents, which is divided into 100 census tracts of approximately 4,000 people each. Each census tract may be described in terms of the aggregate characteristics of its residents: the quality of their housing, educational level, socioeconomic status, ethnic background, family structure, population turnover, sex ratio, age structure, and other characteristics thought to be relevant to the selective use of clinical services.

Thus, the residents of each census tract are described in terms of a series of variables, such as percent living in overcrowded housing, percent over 65 and under 18 years of age, percent families with income under $6,000, percent living alone, percent widowed, percent families with female heads, percent divorced, and so forth. This profile of variables, available from census data, comprise a set of independent variables describing residents of each of the 100 census tracts, which can be used to predict variation in rates of use of clinical services by selected age/sex groups and other categories of users from each of the 100 tracts.

Dependent Variables:
Rates for Clinical Service Use

To estimate rates of service utilization it is necessary to construct a clinical record system which describes the type, frequency, and extent of service rendered to each client, along with selected clinical-historical and sociodemographic variables of value to the clinician, administrator, and epidemiologist-evaluator. Counts from the record system, such as the number of men (age 20−34) using inpatient services during a given time period, can be generated for each census tract and provide the 100 numerators needed to compute a rate variable.

The denominator for such a variable, available from census data, would be the number of men (age 20−34) in each of the 100 census tracts. Basic descriptive statistics on this variable, such as the average rate of inpatient use, the range of rates over the 100 tracts and the variability in rate of use, would provide a basis for speculating about the selective use of inpatient services by this population of young men.

Record System

Development of an effective record system designed for the multiple purpose of administration, clinical service, and evaluation research requires cooperation among representatives of the several disciplines involved, along with consultation from computer scientists and applied measurement experts. The different needs and points of view represented by administrators, clinicians, epidemiologists, and evaluation researchers must be recognized, openly discussed, and ultimately represented in the design of the record system. Both the leadership and authority of key members of the administrative staff are important to the success of the record system.

In making decisions about data to be collected, members of the line clinical staff should be extensively consulted by the research staff so that data useful to the clinician and sufficiently reliable and valid for research purposes are collected. For example, the selection or development of classification systems may become a subject of discussion among the various disciplines. The administrator is held accountable within a legal/fiscal set of standards, the clinician uses a diagnostic classification system compatible with an accepted philosophy of treatment, and the researcher is concerned with the reliability and validity of measures.

A critical but constructive exchange, based on a practical understanding of the current literature relevant to classification systems, should clarify the strengths, weaknesses, and utility of various classification systems as a basis for designing that part of the record system. Researchers should emphasize such issues as lucid definitions, the reliability of ratings, the negative effects of missing data and the need to monitor the accuracy of collected data. The potential value of clearly written summary reports which answer the questions of administrators, clinicians, researchers, and planners should be emphasized as a positive result of accurately collected and appropriately analyzed data sets.

Thus the design, implementation and evaluation of a record system may serve as the beginning of a dialogue among those disciplines involved in the provision and evaluation of clinical services. The continuation of such a dialogue within a clinical service structure could result in the conceptualization and solving of critical problems leading to more effective and responsible service systems. With the current focus on accountability and program evaluation, this cooperative endeavor may become a necessity.

Social Area Characteristics and Rates of Service Use

As previously indicated, two sets of variables—those describing characteristics of census tracts as social areas, and those describing the rates of use by residents of the social areas—may be derived from census data and clinical record systems. Area characteristics were conceived as independent variables; rates of clinical use by categories of area residents as dependent or outcome variables.

Relationships among these variable sets will indicate the extent to which differences among social areas will account for variation in rates of clinical use, answering such questions as:

1. To what extent do residents of low income areas have higher rates of inpatient service use than residents of middle class areas?
2. Is the ethnic composition of social areas related to patterns of use by social area residents?
3. Are the location, quality, and efficiency of the clinical services important determinants of their selective use?
4. Are there sex differences in the use of clinical services, as age is varied?

Combinations of social area characteristics, selected on a hypothetical basis, may be used to understand the relative importance of social area characteristics in predicting patterns of clinical service use. Such multiple correlation are usually in the .7 to .8 range, with indicators of social class and family structure playing the important roles in predicting high rates of use. Results of analyses such as those described would lead to a comprehensive picture of how services are selectively used, inferences about why this is so, and conclusions about whether or not the service delivery system is achieving its purpose and fulfilling its responsibilities.

During the design and implementation of the record system, a parallel study of true prevalence of the catchment area could be planned, profiting, as did the record system, from the exchange between clinicians and epidemiologists. Ideally many of the questions asked in the field study would duplicate those asked of clients of the clinical services, thus making the comparison of data sets possible, as they should be. The completion of a field epidemiological study would be an excellent training exercise for students of the various disciplines of community mental health centers.

Experience in interviewing members of the catchment area population, representing a variety of social class, ethnic, and cultural backgrounds, on their own turf would help the student to understand the influence of social context on behavior, including that of the interviewer. The student could follow the study from the planning-pilot stage through the various steps to the conclusions and implications.

At the completion of the epidemiological field study, results of the two approaches could be compared to see if the clinical services are reaching the high risk areas identified by the field study. Subsequent interviews of the field sample would indicate the rate of use by those with ratings of severe impairment, as illustrated in Dr. Langner's study.

While space precludes the elaboration of a detailed description of how one might proceed, it would seem appropriate, following the above comparisons, to systematically introduce planned innovations in service delivery and to assess their effects in reaching target populations that were identified as underserved by both the results of field epidemiological and social area studies.

This continued examination of the relationship between characteristics of social area residents and their rates of service use should result in the development of effective service delivery and the assessment of the predictive validity of field epidemiological studies, under different service delivery conditions. In accomplishing these purposes, the required exchange among administrators, clinicians, epidemiologists, and evaluators should produce a stimulating educational environment beneficial to both staff and students.

Chapter 3

Evaluation of Community Mental Health Services

Martin Katz (Moderator)

Societal Barriers to Learning: The Community Psychiatry Example

Loren R. Mosher

As a former student of Martin Orne's, I have come to be quite sensitive to the influence of demand characteristics on behavior. When I finally sat down to write this paper, it occurred to me to wonder what the reasons were for the Foundation's choosing this topic at this time. Because I was not privy to the process, or the names of those who influenced it, I was free to fantasize.

It is my presumption, based on the meeting's title: "A *Critical* Appraisal of Community Psychiatry," and because of the title of subsection IV, to which I will address myself: "Re-evaluation of the Theory of Community Psychiatry Based on Relevant Research," that this group has *not* been convened to praise Caesar. Rather, this overwhelmingly white, male, university and governmental elite may have been brought together twenty centuries after Caesar's internment to give senatorial blessing to the assassination of community psychiatry. I am certain the meeting's organizers will deny it. I must wonder, however, given the current political climate, whether community psychiatry is beginning to be set up as a scapegoat for its failure to live up to the exaggerated expectations fostered on its behalf for more than a decade.

The choice of community psychiatry for this role is quite in keeping with its history in this country. That is, 'the community mental health center movement'—which is virtually synonymous with community psychiatry in this country—has been highly politicized from the beginning. The Community Mental Health Center Act of 1963 was largely an outgrowth of, and based on, the report of the Joint

Commission on Mental Illness and Health [1]. In oversimplified terms, this report detailed the bankruptcy and failure of the state hospital system to treat and rehabilitate the mentally ill. It recommended sweeping changes in current and planned state facilities with emphasis to be placed on community-based centers. The Joint Commission foresaw a gradual phasing in of federal subsidies to share the cost of care for the mentally ill ((1) p. xxi).

The process by which the 1963 and 1965 federal legislation came about can be better documented by those closer to it. What happened, whatever the original aims, was the establishment of a federally funded system of CMHCs in competition with (and over the objections of) existing state hospital systems. Thus, rather than evolutionary reform of state mental health programs by use of the federal financial carrot and stick, there was established a revolutionary system of federally financed medical care that essentially by-passed existing state systems and usurped a traditionally state function. It can be seen, in a sense, as the first United States try at federally financed and standardized socialized medicine—but limited to mental illnesses.

It would seem this revolution was allowed to pass Congress and be implemented because it was included among a spate of Kennedy-initiated, but mostly Johnson-passed, "Great Society" programs, acted upon in the sessions that followed President Kennedy's assassination. The irony of setting up a system of socialized medicine, to compete with one whose roots were so firmly embedded in the era of extraordinarily exploitative capitalism and Social Darwinism of the latter half of the nineteenth century, has escaped most people. Unfortunately, this contradiction may have led to much of the difficulty in which community psychiatry finds itself today.

Now, some twelve years after this landmark legislation was passed, we are being asked to "critically appraise" and "re-evaluate" Community Psychiatry. I submit that this can, at best, be the beginning of such a process. Community psychiatry is barely a teenager; it was born into an unfriendly environment; it lived its infancy and latency in a home in which who and what it was to be was variously defined by others; and was surrounded by a social system undergoing unprecedented upheaval. The system's response to these uncertainties was to expect too much of it too soon. So, I must ask, have we been gathered here to begin the process of retreat from community psychiatry and, by so doing, sound its death knell? Are we being asked to sit in judgment of community psychiatry's failures so that its dismantling can be rationalized and justified?

This meeting does occur, after all, at a time when the administration is once again proposing that the federal government get out of the CMHC business. What may even be more important, however, is that many CMHC staffing grants are running out and states are being asked to pick up their tabs. In a bit of Catch–22 so frequently found in our government, Congress has passed the new CMHC bill which requires twelve (rather than five) services, but without extending original staffing grant periods for older CMHCs who wish to comply with the new regulations. Others at this meeting can detail this situation better than I; I raise these issues only to point out that we cannot be asked to be "critical" or to "re-evaluate" independent of the context in which these questions are raised. In the same vein, community psychiatry cannot be viewed independent of the context of its origin, birth, and later development. Leaving aside these contextual considerations would make it much easier to find community psychiatry's deficiencies sufficient to conclude the whole thing was a mistake.

Finally, one other factor that may relate to the demand characteristics of this meeting must be addressed. That is, it occurs at a time when we are witnessing a swing of the pendulum of opinion within our field away from a social model of the causes and treatment of mental disorders to a much more biologically oriented one. This shift is manifest in many ways: more chairs of psychiatry departments are occupied by biologically oriented psychiatrists, more biologically oriented research is funded now, clinical psychiatrists more and more rely on psychopharmacological treatment, and so forth. As many of community psychiatry's assumptions are at variance with the disease in the individual model espoused by most biologically oriented psychiatrists, this meeting may be asking us to criticize and re-evaluate (devalue?) community psychiatry so as to provide impetus for the pendulum to swing even further away from the social model.

I will be critical of community psychiatry's lack of true innovation and evaluation efforts. However, I hope to bring what might be termed a Mark Antony perspective to this critique. I shall appear to conform to the demand characteristics of this meeting and come to bury community psychiatry, not to praise it. Yet, I believe in so doing it will be obvious that its deficiencies are explicable and its contributions praiseworthy indeed.

BARRIERS TO THE EVALUATION IN COMMUNITY PSYCHIATRY

Shifting Definitions of Concepts

The task I agreed to assume here was the *re-evaluation* of theoretical assumptions of community psychiatry based on research. Yet, as I began to prepare material for this paper, it became clear that there was no clear, consistent, well articulated set of assumptions that comprise a testable theory. Furthermore, most of its assumptions were not evaluated prior to implementation. Therefore, re-evaluation is impossible. We are left with attempting to evaluate certain of its assumptions (not a theory) for the first time; for example, continuity of care. Yet this assumption is difficult to subject to rigorous evaluation because of differences in the way it can be defined. It may mean anything from a team's being responsible for the care of an individual patient wherever he is in the system, to one where the patient is shifted from place to place within the system, with continuity meaning nothing more than telephone notification of transfer.

Medical Domination

One assumption of community psychiatry with which I have been particularly intrigued is its espousal of local wards (usually in general hospitals) to the wards of state hospitals. It is notable that a system originally set up as a competitive alternative to state hospitals has done so little to define the breadth and limitations of possible alternatives to hospitalization. The Joint Commission's report clearly mandates the use of alternatives to hospitalization wherever feasible. Although CMHCs use inpatient care less often than do state hospitals, they have not committed themselves to the development of non-hospital alternatives.

For me, at least, these alternatives should be of central concern to a true *community* psychiatry. They should be new types of programs really in the community—that is, with their participants having ongoing interaction with the neighborhoods within which they are embedded. Instead, community psychiatry has defined inpatient care in general hospitals as community care but rejects inpatient care in state hospitals—with precious little data to support the notion that well staffed general hospital wards are better than equally well staffed state hospitals. Given their situation, this is not difficult to explain: that is, for the most part, doctors are in power in CMHCs. As the implementation of community psychiatry was new to everyone in 1964, doctors who were in charge modified slightly what they knew and applied it under the new community psychiatry rubric. As others have already pointed out [2], it has come to be business-as-usual with a new label.

As the original law required an inpatient service, there was little impetus *not* to use it with seriously disordered individuals (e.g., functional psychotics in particular). What has evolved over the past decade or so is a *belief* that short stays in community hospital wards are better than longer stays in state hospitals. However, the critical experiment—short-stay general hospital versus longer-stay state hospital where staffing is equivalent—has not been done. The recent study of Glick et al. [3] comes closest to addressing this question. Unfortunately, short stays seem to be dictated more by politics and economics than by the belief that they are actually "better" [4]. In fact, they eventuate in the revolving door phenomenon because they do not allow sufficient time for recovery of psychosocial functioning (rather than symptom remission). They may actually turn out to be economically unsound over the longer term [5] because schizophrenia's major cost to society is from loss of productivity—*not* the direct cost of treatment.

In addition, if research did not demonstrate that general hospital wards were superior to state hospital care, the entire CMHC program, and with it the powerful bureaucracies developed to administer it, would be threatened. This situation naturally creates a need within these bureaucracies not to know, a need which cannot be overcome in the absence of strong outside incentives.

Absence of Incentives for Evaluation

Evaluation is really a form of organized, formalized, externally visible self-criticism. As clinicians know, self-criticism and accepting criticisms of others is easier when we feel relatively secure. Needless to say, the early days of community psychiatry were not secure. There were few models for CMHCs available. What would constitute a CMHC was poorly defined in the law, and the National Institute of Mental Health was uncertain as to how it would define this new offspring.

One way of dealing with the uncertainty in such situations is to arbitrarily define goals and pursue them with evangelistic fervor. This may be one way early entrants in the CMHC derby got programs started. Needless to say, religions like these are difficult to subject to objective scientific evaluation. The internal reward system for new CMHCs was based on service delivered, smoothly functioning clinical teams, and group cohesiveness to a common goal. For administrators, it was program expansion, development of new services, and finding the money to support them. Research was not required, nor was it a source of significant prestige or power. There was no special federal research carrot offered. Program evaluation research was not required by the original law. Given this context, it is no wonder so little research was done.

In 1969, NIMH received authority from the CMHC Act to conduct program evaluation studies. In 1970, authority was given the Secretary of HEW to use up to 1 percent of the annual appropriation for evaluation. Yet, program evaluation was still not required of CMHC grant recipients. Many CMHC people will say they have program evaluation built into their systems. However, this is almost always confined to resource utilization (number of visits, days of inpatient care, etc.). Unfortunately, evaluation that does not include the study of patient outcome is of only limited utility for feeding back to programs so that they can be modified in response to the evaluation data. Hence, the basic need not to know is not violated by this type of evaluation.

Interestingly, the "1 percent money" made available by the 1969 and 1970 amendments is administered in Washington, D.C. For the most part, this money is not given out via the traditional NIH/NIMH peer review process. Thus, the protection from politicalization inherent in peer review is much less true of the 1 percent money. So, despite this new emphasis on program evaluation, there was relatively little impetus for *individual* CMHCs to start their own evaluation programs. In fact, this 1 percent money might have had negative consequences for research. It is only human for CMHC administrators to regard being researched by *outsiders* as threatening, resulting in noncooperation.

Their perception is, of course, accurate. Evaluation research provides data on which to base decisions about program maintenance, expansion, or contraction based on effectiveness. While the centralized evaluation coffers grew, the principal NIMH Branch funding evaluation via the usual peer review process has had an essentially level budget since 1969. This represents a more than 25 percent decline in real dollars over the 1969–75 period. In practice, this meant it was even more difficult for individual CMHCs to obtain program evaluation money.

Shifting Demands

The evaluation of psychiatric treatment, except for psychopharmacological agents, is notoriously complex, arduous, and difficult. To attempt a study of patient outcomes (*not* resource utilization— essentially a bookkeeping operation) requires a sophisticated, dedicated, stable research team with good knowledge of the day-to-day workings of the facility. They must be in close touch with the front line clinical personnel and responsive to their needs so their cooperation—without which the study cannot be done—can be maintained. The research team leader must command the respect and absolute support of the administration.

Even if all these conditions are met, the problems inherent in this

type of research may be insuperable. For example, patient characteristics are very heterogeneous; treatments given are heterogeneous;
and responses to a given treatment, even with similar patients, may
vary widely. So, large samples, studied over relatively long periods
of time, may be necessary. Yet Americans are very mobile, making
followup a formidable obstacle. Shifts in the political and economic
picture outside the facility will result in unanticipated program
changes. This is what drives experimentalists wild. CMHC programs
just won't hold still to be studied. An open, socially oriented ward
will be changed into a locked medical model one with a change of
psychiatrists in charge. A researcher studying outcomes in patients
from that ward must divide his subjects into two cohorts; social and
medical. Given the other difficulties noted above, it may make it
impossible to draw any firm conclusions, despite his best efforts.

IMPLEMENTATION BARRIERS

In the previous section I attempted to define a variety of contextual
barriers to evaluation research in community psychiatry. Based on
that discussion, I am amazed that evaluation is done at all! But how
can community psychiatry's failure to implement relatively well
studied established-as-effective programs be explained? I will use
three examples from what seems to be an underemphasized aspect
of community psychiatry, to which I alluded earlier—the development of alternatives to hospitalization for very distrubed individuals.
    During the 1960s three groups of investigators studied very dif-
ferent alternatives to hospitalization for three different types of
patients. Fairweather et al. [6] developed a community "lodge" for
a heterogenous (mostly psychotic) group of Veterans Administration
Hospital patients. Pasamanick and his co-workers [7] used home care
with visiting nurses and medication to avoid hospitalization in a
group of married schizophrenic women. And Langsley et al. [8]
studied family crisis intervention in a heterogenous group of acutely
disturbed patients deemed in need of hospitalization.
    The results indicated, in each instance, that on most measures of
outcome the experimental groups fared better than comparable controls. Yet, for the most part, only Fairweather's results have been
fairly widely utilized [9]. This is, at least in part, the result of his
having received an NIMH dissemination and utilization grant. At last
count there were 25 to 30 lodges in existence in twelve to fifteen
different locations—mostly associated with state hospitals. The findings of the other two studies have resulted in some new programs in
some places; neither investigator could say how often. Neither have

been subjected to experimental replication, which is one indication of scientific interest at least. The state in which Pasamanick's program was initiated and studied chose not to support it after the research terminated.

It is both hazardous and difficult to assess retrospectively the reasons why these seemingly useful new approaches were not widely implemented in a program whose legislation, at least, was revolutionary. However, a brief discussion of the problems these programs might create for CMHCs may be illuminating. This discussion is based in large part on our experience with trying to sell a philosophically similar alternative to hospitalization to established CMHC programs. The barriers are not necessarily listed in order of importance.

Business as Usual

As I noted previously, this means the treatment of seriously disturbing behavior on wards, in places called hospitals, with attendant medically dominated hierarchies. Data from all programs (the three mentioned above plus our own) indicate that at least *some* patients are better treated in nonhospital residential settings. Successful implementation of any of these programs would require major changes in concept, attitude, and practice, especially among psychiatrists. The medical model, while heuristically valuable, has some difficulty giving adequate credence to families and social environments in the production and course of psychiatric disorder. Treating individual patients in his office or in the hospital is more consonant with most psychiatrist's concepts and training, than is the case with home or other social environment centered treatment.

The community psychiatry movement has, for the most part, been medicalized. A new bureaucracy has been created with trappings appropriate to it; wards, clinics, offices, administrators, case conferences, etc. For example, the vast majority of CMHC inpatient services are wards in general hospitals. I have come more and more to see how bureaucratization is, in fact, antithetical to real helping. I submit that the control of the CMHC program by the relatively conservative medical profession and the bureaucracy that grew to administer it has been a major barrier to both evaluation and innovation in it.

Threats to Professionalism

All four of these hospital alternative programs used relatively small numbers (or none in one case) of doctors or PhDs as primary therapists. In fact, one measure of success in Fairweather's program was when the last professional ceased contact with the lodge and it became a totally autonomous unit. It is difficult, indeed, to imagine salaried professionals, whose power comes in part from their being necessary for the operation of programs, welcoming with open arms new programs that do not require their services. Widespread establishment of these alternatives could, carried to their logical conclusion, result in a major shift in the locus of power, control, and responsibility in the mental health field. Needless to say, this revolutionary proletarianization will be resisted by those currently in power.

Lack of Incentives for Innovation. Unfortunately, the CMHC law does not require creation of, or research on, new *types* of services. This is not to take away from its important role in changing patterns of facility use and bringing mental health care closer to many people. Here again, the constantly shifting demands (usually politically and economically determined) to which many CMHCs are subjected does not create a fertile soil for the propagation or study of locally created innovative programs. In this situation, external rewards become key and there are few. The 1975 law does remedy this to some extent but its potential for significant impact, given the problems with it I mentioned earlier, remains open to serious question.

Public Uninterest. In 1972, there were more than 2.7 million admissions to all types of mental health facilities [10]. Patients who received only outpatient care from a private psychiatrist are not included in this count. It never ceases to amaze me how, when somewhere between 1.5 and 2 percent of the United States population receives mental health care in any given year (an even higher percentage of families are affected), there is so little consumerism or pressure brought to bear on legislators demanding better and more equitable care. Can we conclude they are satisfied with what they are receiving? I doubt, it, when nearly 600,000 of these admissions are to state hospitals. In our own survey of patient and family satisfaction with treatment received in the CMHC which serves as our control facility, we found that about 90 percent of patients and 80 percent of families were dissatisfied with the care they received.

I believe a variety of factors are operating to prevent patients and families from forming pressure groups. There is space to mention only a few. They protest little for at least three reasons. First, persons from the lower social classes are overrepresented among mental patients. Their previous experiences of powerlessness to resist demands for submission to authority lead them to accept, relatively unquestioningly, what the *medical* system offers. Their alternatives are limited. It is a basically "take it or leave it" system. Second, as a group, people who get labeled "mentally ill" are deviant from society's norms and generally less competent (at least in terms of ability to work productively) than the other members of society; ergo, it is more difficult for them both to organize consumer groups and to be taken seriously. Third, patients and their families generally want to keep their madness (if not the madpersons to themselves these days), safely hidden in the closet.

What about the general public? Why is there so little real interest in the mentally ill? At least two reasons are operating. First, with the exception of drugs, there are not great corporate profits to be made from mental illness. Like all human service industries, it is labor—intensive. Second, although better hidden today than before, much of the public fears the mentally ill and would prefer *not* to have to deal with them on a day-by-day basis. I believe this public attitude is a major source of difficulty for community psychiatry, which asks the public to tolerate deviance in its midst. There are many recent examples of this basic mistrust of the mentally ill making itself felt. The Long Island city that passed an ordinance to bar ex-patients from residing there is one example.

In the 1970s we are witnessing a reaction to the social upheavals of the 1960s. Part of this response is a lowering of tolerance for deviance that cannot help but present problems for community-based programs. This is not a climate in which innovation, change, and open-minded seeking of better solutions to persistent problems is facilitated, much less demanded. Quite the contrary, the public demands a return to what is known and safe. Community psychiatry is responding to this demand by returning to traditional medical views of madness.

A Case Study of "Community" Psychiatry

In May 1971, Alma Menn and I began a comparative outcome study of two matched cohorts of first-break, unmarried schizophrenic patients between 16 and 30 years of age, deemed in need of hospitalization and followed for two years. Both experimental and control patients were obtained from a large screening facility (600 new patients a month) which is part of a community mental health center. Patients who met the research criteria were assigned on a consecutively admitted, space available basis to either the experimental or control group. The control patients were admitted to the wards of the community mental health center, where they received "usual" treatment. Experimental patients, on the other hand, were treated at Soteria, a comfortably 16-room home in the San Francisco Bay area. Both groups were assessed on the same battery of tests.

The CMHC serves part of a sprawling Bay Area suburban/urban county containing about one million persons. It is divided into five catchment areas, each served by its own regional facility. The CMHC that serves as the control facility in the study is located roughly in the county's geographic center. Its own catchment area has a wide socioeconomic spread but its clientele are mostly lower middle class. It is unique in the county because it has the only locked wards and twenty-four-hour psychiatric emergency service. It also houses the mental health administration for the entire county. The county mental health chief, a psychiatrist, has been in his job for over ten years. His budget is about $13 million per year, comprised of a mix of state, county, and federal funds. He answers to the county board of supervisors and a mental health advisory board. Most of the county's money is spent via contractual arrangements with private agencies which provide services for the county. This report will focus principally on the central center's inpatient services.

In 1971, the center had one 30-bed, open unit in the adjacent county hospital. Bed costs were $90 per day. Because the state's formula for funding county programs included a penalty for using state hospital beds, the county began renovating a medical ward to become another 30-bed inpatient unit. They anticipated this would decrease their use of the nearby state hospital.

In July 1971, just two months after our study began, the state proposed closing the mental illness sections of the nearby state hospital. This was a combined consolidation/economy move. The state closed admissions to the hospital in November 1971. For the next three months, until their second ward was ready, the county had to send all excess hospital patients to another state hospital 100 miles north. Their second ward opened in February 1972 with high expectations. The best of the former state hospital staff moved there (there is a 1.5/1 staff/patient ratio), a new, young, dynamic ward chief was appointed, and university residents soon began to be trained there. The number of admissions soon reached 250 per month, and they have remained relatively stable since.

For two years, beginning in the spring of 1972, through the same time in 1974, both wards had stable leadership and were allowed to pretty much plan and run their own programs. On one of them a "social" model was implemented, with paraprofessionals sharing in the responsibility, power, and authority. The other developed a doctor oriented, traditional medical model program. Beginning in the spring of 1974, increasing pressures were placed on the wards to decrease length of stays and use less bed days in the state hospital, as each of these cost the county significantly. By this time bed costs were $140 per day so the three-day rise in average length of stay, from five to eight days, that occurred over the previous year raised inpatient costs by more than 1/3 above original estimates. In addition, the county had been sending between 20 and 30 patients per month to the state hospital; in California, the cost of their care is subtracted from the state's 90 percent payment to the county.

This change in length of stay and increased use of state hospital occurred despite both units' philosophies being focused on triage, crisis intervention, rapid tranquilization, and placement of patients in other parts of the county's treatment network as rapidly as possible—with the result that many patients fall through the "cracks." These economically engendered administrative pressures resulted in the resignation of both ward chiefs and a decline in morale of the staff, who now felt, realistically, that economic needs were not compatible with their patients' treatment needs.

Between January and July 1975, a sociologist, Holly Wilson, PhD, went onto these wards to describe them. As a former nurse, she is uniquely qualified to describe hospital ward processes. Her report is based on 120 hours of participant observation on the ward, which included time spent on all shifts, attendance at all meetings, review of all the ward's written documents (e.g., guidelines for medical coverage, nursing notes), and informal interviews with all types of staff. She describes the ward's primary overall functioning as a "dispatching process" with a variety of subprocesses as follows.

1. *Patching.* Staff's initial contact with patients often revolves around the imposition of a variety of behavioral controls such as use of seclusion rooms, mechanical restraints, verbal instructions, and particularly heavy doses of psychotropic medications such as Haldol, Prolixin, or Thorazine. In essence, violent, out of control, or inappropriately bizarre patients are *patched together* by subduing their socially unacceptable symptoms as quickly as possible.

2. *Medical screening.* Because the psychiatric dispatching process (a term used to encompass the multiple, complex operations employed for "processing patients through" a clearing house model of care) takes place in a "medical" setting under the direction of physicians for the most part, a standardized routine of physical testing and diagnostic procedures is immediately initiated for all new admissions. These procedures include a physical exam, blood work, urinalysis, E.E.G., and a selected variety of others. Such screening also serves as an information gathering strategy in that on occasion a patient's psychiatric problem is discovered to be a consequence of a medical or physiological disorder. Properties of this process of screening are that it is extremely time-consuming for staff, that it requires accurate and proper completion of a multitude of requisitions and

forms, and that it is rigidly imposed, even though a patient who is readmitted may have undergone the same screening process within the same week.

3. *Piecing together a story.* Proportionately speaking, the most staff time and energy is devoted to this dimension of the dispatching process. In order to make subsequent decisions about distributing a patient to the appropriate aftercare placement, as well as the more immediate decision of which course of medications to begin, a diagnosis must be made. Thus, information gathering and intelligence operations consume staff's focus during the first 72 hours of a patient's confinement. The interaction of staff attempting to sleuth out and uncover information about a patient in order to engage in fate-making decisions, with patients who are attempting to cover up what they believe is damaging data about themselves, constitutes another key focus for staff/patient contact. The major modalities for this contact are the "Group Intake Interview" wherein a newly admitted patient is confronted by a group of staff in an interview room and questioned, and the "Second-hand Report" where bits and pieces of data are passed along from shift to shift verbally and on the patient's chart and then used to make generalizations about the patient. Properties of this process are its preconceived tendency, a reliance on speculations which easily become "truth," and the trickery involved in "finding things out."

4. *Labeling and sorting.* Once there is sufficient data to justify some decisions, patients are stamped with a psychiatric label. For the most part, patients in the study setting fell into the following diagnostic categories: schizophrenic, manic-depressive, alcohol or drug abuse, or violent character disorder of some type. *Labeling* acts as a key in deciding which medications to order and which aftercare placements to begin exploring. It also provides staff with an additional source of control in their dealings with patients, for with diagnoses comes an increased sense of being able to predict patient behavior and the ability to deal with patient communications and behaviors as typifications—"That's her hysterical personality coming out; those are just delusions, etc."

5. *Distributing.* The official goal of Community Mental Health legislation in California also includes a goal of moving mentally ill persons back into "the community" as rapidly as possible. Yet, psychiatric professionals in the study setting are constantly balancing this mandate against their perceived mandate to act as protectors of society and their patients. Consequently, staff act as fate-makers by distributing their "charges" to one of a variety of placement options for followup and aftercare. A property of the distributing stage of dispatching is its revolving door nature. Many of the setting's patients are "old familiars," who periodically rotate through the study setting and back out again. A number of patients are *tracked* by community liaison workers which contributes additional data taken into account when distributing decisions are made. Reports include that one aftercare facility or another "won't take her back again" so the options become limited by virtue of exhausting some of them over time.

The above conceptualization of "usual psychiatric care" in the study setting conveys, I hope, the complex nature of the psychiatric decision making and deposition process that goes on. Consequences of these operations include: (1) A very hectic and busy pace of work for staff while the hours "drift by" for patients. (2) A low accessibility of staff for patients—sitting and talking with patients has very low priority in view of all the tasks that must be accomplished. (3) A substitution of technology for potential face-to-face contacts (e.g., there's a mechanical cigarette lighter on the wall to discourage patients from bothering busy staff for lights, medications are announced over a loud speaker instead of passed out by a nurse who seeks out patients around the ward, etc.). (4) Staff spend the majority of their time in interaction with other staff—in report, team meetings, intake interviews, and other meetings. (This observation differed on the two wards with more staff/patient contact on Ward I, in ritualized formats such as "anger group," "feelings group," etc., but these contacts were low on spontaneity, low on openness, and high on superficiality and control.). (5) Staff are the constants on the units with patients only passing through, thus a lot of energy is devoted to intrastaff conflict, problems, and the distribution of labor. (6) Most staff have a lot of integrity about their work— their value systems are relatively congruent with conventional psychiatric and medical model explanations of madness.

Not long after Dr. Wilson completed her observations, a new crisis occurred: a strike of all county employees. The professionals were left to manage the wards, patients were discharged or sent to the state hospital, police served as ward staff, and everyone saw it as 'an awful experience.' The mental health administration's response after the strike was settled was to close one ward and substitute a ten-bed holding unit. This lasted ten weeks until the ward was reopened, but now the facility had 42 instead of 60 beds. One psychiatrist was given charge of both wards. A strict medical model was now to be adhered to, as it is "most efficient," with authority resting at the top of the hierarchy, rule by edict, no attention to the feelings or needs of staff, no responsibility in paraprofessional hands, and so on.

Professtional staff are now leaving. The paraprofessionals' morale is lower than ever but they feel they cannot leave as there are few other jobs available in the area. For the administration, the strike was not all bad. By decreasing the number of beds they could decrease their staff costs and force even shorter lengths of stay (i.e., same number of admissions to fewer beds requires fewer average number of days in hospital to keep up with the demand). There is little apparent concern for what it means in terms of the further bureaucratization and concentration of power, authority, and responsibility at the top of the hierarchy. In my estimation, it cannot bode well for quality of patient care.

In this example, I have said little about research. The CMHC itself is doing none, other than keeping the utilization figures required by the county and state administrations. From the beginning they have agreed to participate in and cooperate with our research, yet on a day-to-day basis, holding their cooperation has been difficult. This is the result of a variety of factors: Our research tends to be viewed as alien since it is not conducted by members of their staff. Their leadership allows it, but is not committed to it. Their staff are already so overburdened it is difficult for them to even think about our research needs. Their staff turnover makes continuity of the research needs in their consciousness difficult for us to maintain. Finally, our experimental facility is almost exactly the opposite of their ward's organization: there is minimal bureaucracy and hierarchy, the pace is leisurely, human concerns are more important than administrative ones, power and responsibility are shared widely.

As it embodies much of what they would like but cannot get in the CMHC setting, many staff there feel frustrated and envious of us. These emotions are not very conducive to whole hearted cooperation. We have made a variety of attempts to overcome these problems, such as hiring a member of their staff to do our evaluations, giving them feedback on the research results, conducting staff training for them, etc. This has had only minimal impact. Without the strong commitment of their leadership, the institution's bureaucracy stands very much in the way of recruiting their active participation in research.

This is one example of present-day "community" psychiatry. The facility and its staff must attempt to reconcile a number of contradictory expectations: protect the community but return its rejects to it as rapidly as possible; give high quality care but do it at low cost; show that what you are doing is worthwhile but without the necessary resources and expertise. They are in a classic no-win situation. Only major shifts in attitude in the community, and in the county and state administration could allow them to carry out the aims of true community psychiatry.

QUO VADIS?

It is often said that community psychiatry has taken patients out of the back wards of state hospitals and put them into one-person back wards in the community. Please remember though, that a person in the community is in control of his own destiny, is not locked in, wears his own clothes, has privacy, can make use of whatever recreation the community offers, can drink and have sex with another consenting adult without fear of reprisal.

Increased reproductive rates in madpersons are viewed with alarm by some who fear the gene pool for madness is being increased. Responsibility of this is generally attributed to the community psychiatry movement. I can only applaud; it is high time we gave up nineteenth century Social Darwinism in favor of a new humanism. In fact, higher reproductive rates among schizophrenics may actually be increasing the society's potential for creativity.

It is said that the high current readmission rates are evidence of community psychiatry's failure. I believe it is evidence of their success in making inpatient care accessible, and of short duration, to avoid the adverse effects of too long hospitalizations. Although I personally disagree with the mindless use of short stays, the hopefulness, positive expectations, and willingness to take risks inherent in any program that emphasizes short hospital stays are tremendously important forces for the good with patients.

Some professionals complain that the community psychiatry movement has resulted in role diffusion and confusion as to who is supposed to do what, when, and where. As a professional, I have gradually come to realize how hiding behind my professionalism can impede my ability to be helpful to another human being. What is called role diffusion by some I would see as legitimization of the notion that, if they want to, human beings can be of help to each other as equals. For me, this is a highly laudable trend, which should be extended even further until such time as we have a community psychiatry which fits Almond's [11] definition of "communitas—a sense of being part of a group of essentially equal members who are important to one another."

It is said that CMHCs do not like to treat seriously disturbed persons. It is often implied that *they* are responsible when a current or former patient makes sensational headlines. How many members of this audience treat psychotics on a day-to-day basis? If by not treating them the CMHCs are allowing more psychotics to run free in the community, I can only say, at least they are more true to Hippocrates in "doing no harm" than is the case when madpersons are locked up in distant, inhuman state hospitals. For me, the occasional untoward event is far preferable to the loss of freedom necessary to really "protect" society from the possibility of mental patients doing something criminal. In fact, Brill's data [12] indicate that ex-mental patients do not commit more crimes than the average.

By resisting society's unrealistic demand for safety from madpersons, community psychiatry can be a potent force for the preservation of freedom for all of us. It is important that we all resist the temptation to hold a system or a bureaucracy responsible for that which we disapprove. Individuals are responsible—not bureaucracies. These contributions are very important. For me, community psychiatry has had to overcome such great difficulties that I am surprised at the number of contributions it has made. Each should be carried further. Critics should not be allowed to force a retreat.

In conclusion, looking back over what I have said, I have to ask myself if my assessment is a eulogy or a progress report? I wish I knew. At worst, if my assessment of the direction of movement at this time is correct it may be a tombstone inscription written in advance of actually dying. Although the term community psychiatry may survive, the opportunity for real change in the ways in which help is given and received may have eluded us.

It is tempting to choose one isolated element from the many I have described and ascribe to it a primary role in community psychiatry's having blown its big chance. Scapegoating the bureaucratization or the lack of a proper definition of "community" in human interactive terms or the conservative medical profession, would be an easy way out. I believe the flaw is in the fabric of the entire society— and, as such, in each of us as well. We cannot reasonably expect the so-called "mentally ill" to manifest "communitas" when the rest of society does not. We have the senatorial elite and the mass of ordinary citizenry; there are the exploiters and the exploited; the powerful and the powerless; the rich and the poor. Human considerations are secondary to economic ones.

I need not bore you with the long list of inequities and incongruities in this society. We all seem to choose not to acknowledge them, for to do so would mean we would feel individually responsible for doing something about them. In a sense, we all choose not to know. Being human, we seek a means of shifting responsibility for not knowing to something or someone outside ourselves. How can we hold community psychiatry responsible for not knowing and not being innovative, when it is really only following society's dictates? A true, knowing, and innovative community psychiatry can hardly be expected to develop until we are all committed to knowing and can accept responsibility for doing something about the contradictions and inequities in our society.

Ethnicity and the Delivery of Mental Health Services

Gary L. Tischler

A basic social policy objective of the federal community mental health center program is to insure the availability of mental health services in the community to all residents of a defined geographic area called the catchment " . . . regardless of age, sex, race, creed, color, national origin, diagnostic category, voluntary or involuntary status, or ability to pay" [1]. Few would deny the merit of this objective. As Mechanic [2] suggests, however, the reach of social policy may well extend beyond the limits of knowledge and technology.

This is particularly true where intervention strategies are based upon a single theory or a set of theories that have only achieved a modest level of confirmation. Under such circumstances, ideologies and ideologues abound. The idealogues proselytize their ideology. The proselytes band together as a constituency and attempt to transform their belief system into an action system. The end result of this beneficence may come to take the form of social policy.

Far be it for me to suggest that this is what has happened. Rather, my concern is with a tendency to assume that the quality of services rendered and the benefit derived from care are corollaries of accessibility and availability. With this in mind, I would like to discuss a series of studies that focus upon various aspects of the relationship betwen ethnicity and the delivery of mental health services.

STUDY 1: ETHNICITY, PSYCHOLOGICAL IMPAIRMENT AND THE DEMAND FOR CARE

The first study addresses the relationship between ethnicity, the need for care, and the demand for service. Data were available from a random household survey of the catchment that was conducted by Myers, Lindenthal, and Pepper [3]. They measured the mental health status of survey participants using an instrument developed by Macmillan and later modified by Gurin and associates [4, 5]. Previous research indicated that relatively low Gurin scores identified individuals with major psychological problems. For this study, the sample was dichotomized in order to distinguish persons exhibiting "high symptom levels" from all other survey respondents. This group was then defined as "the impaired survey subsample." It consisted of 16 percent of the survey population.

To determine the relationship between ethnicity, psychological impairment, and service utilization, age specific comparisons were made of the proportion of nonwhites in the impaired vs. nonimpaired survey subsamples, in the full survey vs. patient populations, and in the impaired survey subsample vs. the patient population. As Table 3—1 indicates, the proportion of nonwhites is significantly greater in the impaired vs. nonimpaired survey subsamples and in the patient vs. full survey populations. No significant difference is noted between the impaired survey subsample and the patient population. These findings apply to all age groups.

The results demonstrate an association between ethnicity and the distribution of symptomatology in the community, with proportionally greater representation of nonwhites in the impaired survey subsample. While nonwhites are "overrepresented" as patients in relation to the community-at-large, the proportion of nonwhite patients does not differ significantly from the proportion of nonwhites in the impaired community subsample.

Where high facility utilization mirrors the distribution of symptomatology in the community, a true concordance exists between the need for care and demand for service. If one accepts Andersen's premise that the equitable distribution of services occurs when the primary determinants of utilization are perceived need and evaluated need, the demonstrated concordance provides presumptive evidence of basic equity in the service system being studied [6].

STUDY 2: ETHNIC DIFFERENTIALS IN THE DISTRIBUTION OF DEMAND

The overall demand, however, is distributed among four major organizational elements. These include community satellites, ambulatory care services, full—partial hospitalization, and specialty programs. Since the specialty programs have as their target populations either substance abusers or Spanish-Americans, one would anticipate a bias in demand favoring ethnic minorities. Similarly, the inpatient—partial hospitalization programs should draw their patients from the more

Table 3–1. Ethnicity, the Need for Care, and the Demand for Service

Age Groups	Population at Large	Patient Population	Survey Subsample	
			Impaired	Nonimpaired
Ethnicity % nonwhite				
20–29	24	36	35	21
30–49	19	34	34	17
50+	6	12	11	4

Chi-square values, nonimpaired vs. impaired subsamples, significant at the 5% level.
Chi-square values, impaired survey subsample vs. patient population, nonsignificant.
Chi-square values, patient population vs. population at large, significant at the 5% level.

166 New Trends of Psychiatry in the Community

severely impaired segments of the community-at-large. Given the distribution of symptomatology in the community, one would expect higher utilization of these services by nonwhites. The ambulatory care and community satellite programs, however, are multiservice entities. Their armamentaria include an array of social services as well as mental health evaluation and treatment services.

As Table 3−2 indicates, the demand made upon this service constellation by nonwhites occurs at a rate more than twofold that exhibited by whites living within the catchment: 26.8/1000 versus 12.5/1000. Ethnic differentials in demand emerge only in relation to the full−partial hospitalization and specialty programs. Nonsignificant differences are noted for the ambulatory care and community satellite programs. Thus the magnitude of the original difference in demand emerges as a function of the performance of two service elements.

STUDY 3: ETHNIC DIFFERENTIALS IN PATTERNS OF CARE

The existence of ethnic differentials in the distribution of demand suggests that a more detailed inquiry into patterns of utilization is in order. To accomplish this, a utilization profile was developed. The profile consists of three indices:

1. The Service Use Rate (SUR) represents an unduplicated count of all additions to a particular unit (admissions, readmissions, transfers in) during a twelve-month period and is expressed as a rate per thousand. It is intended to provide a more comprehensive statement concerning overall utilization than could be obtained from just surveying admissions and readmissions. This is particularly true of units which act primarily as receiving rather than admitting services.

Table 3−2. Ethnic Differentials in the Utilization of Major Service Elements

| | Ethnicity | |
Service Element	White	Nonwhite
Specialty programs[a]	1.2	9.3
Full/Partial hospitalization[a]	1.8	7.5
Ambulatory care[b]	6.5	7.0
Community satellites[b]	3.0	3.0

[a]Z Scores are significant at the .002 level.
[b]Z Scores are nonsignificant.

2. The Discharge Index (DI) is that proportion of all patients receiving treatment during a twelve-month period (admissions, transfers in, patients on books at the start of the fiscal year) who were terminated during that time. A high index score indicates that the unit acts as a final path in a patient's treatment career in the organization.

3. The Retention Index (RI) provides a rough measure of the tendency of a particular unit to retain people in treatment. It reflects that proportion of the overall user pool receiving care during a twelve-month period who remain on service at the end of this time period.

For the present analyses, the major service elements were subdivided into their component parts (Table 3–3). Ethnic differentials in overall utilization, as reflected by the Service Use Rate, were noted in relation to all elements of the specialty and full–partial hospitalization programs. No significant differences emerged for the elements of the ambulatory care program or for the community satellite program. In relation to the character of care, however, the biases did not invariably favor ethnic minorities. The medical maintenance–resocialization unit is primarily an after care program serving a population of chronic psychotics who have experienced multiple hospitalizations. While the SUR was similar, nonwhite patients were more likely to be discharged and less likely to be retained on service during a twelve month period.

Similarly, nonwhite patients of the psychotherapy unit were less likely to remain in continued care, despite the fact that a substantial portion of this unit's activity is devoted to the provision of long term care. Conversely, the ambulatory services offered by the community satellite programs and specialty programs (excepting the drug dependence unit), show service biases in the character of care favoring nonwhites.

While there is strong representation of ethnic minorities on all service elements, the analyses suggest that it is possible to structure a service system so as to maximize accessibility, while simultaneously developing service subsystems that deal more selectively with certain problems and population subgroups. These subsystems may operate differentially either to counter or to support social policy objectives. Indeed, they may be constructed so that barriers to service that formerly existed at an entry level are moved deeper into an organization's infrastructure, where they are less visible.

Table 3–3.   Ethnic Differentials in Patterns of Care

	Service Use Rate			Discharge Index		Retention Index	
	White		Nonwhite	White	Nonwhite	White	Nonwhite
Ambulatory Care							
Evaluation/Brief treatment	6.1		6.6	46	53	11	8
Psychotherapies	3.5	***	3.3	38	45	35	18
Medication Maintenance/Resocialization	1.1		1.0	17	36	70	52
Specialty Programs							
Drug dependence	1.7	***	9.6	49	40	23	24
Other	0.8	***	5.3	33	29	51	74
Community Satellites	3.3		3.9	50	32	45	55
Full/Partial Hospitalization							
Day hospital	0.8	*****	1.8	29	45	6	10
Inpatient	3.3	***	9.3	33	39	6	6

Chi-square values significant at the 5% level.

***   Z Scores significant at .002 level.
*****   Z Scores significant at .05   level.

STUDY 4: ETHNICITY AND THE QUALITY OF CARE

The analytic procedures used previously represent mechanisms for identifying biases in the delivery of mental health services. These may be entry, distributive, or performance biases. Their presence merely indicates that differentials exist in terms of who is served or the character of care provided. Even where the biases conform with broad social policy objectives, as was generally the case in the present study, further investigation is required to determine whether observed differentials are consistent with "good" as opposed to "bad" clinical practice.

To explore the issue of the relationship between the quality of service rendered and differentials in patterns of care, recourse was made to a criteria oriented approach for evaluating the care giving process [7, 8]. The approach begins with the formulation of normative criteria of service appropriateness and adequacy by panels of expert clinicians. By appropriateness, I mean that admission to treatment is justified by and consistent with the presenting problem; by adequacy, that treatment unfolds in an orderly sequence and, in its conduct, conforms with established standards of excellence within the field. The criteria are then transformed into an abstract format, which enables a nonclinician to make yes-no discriminations concerning the character of care on the basis of a review of the patient's record. An example of the transformation is provided in Figure 3—1.

The record review by the nonclinician is a screening device intended to identify instances where card does not conform with preestablished criteria. When such a determination is made, the record is forwarded to a clinician reviewer. A general question is posed in relation to the category of care being queried: "Was the medication adequate? Explain." The clinician reviewer examines the entire clinical record; makes a judgment as to whether each issue raised is indicative of adequate, adequate but unusual, or inadequate care; and explains the basis for that judgment. In addition, the clinician reviewer also renders a global judgment concerning the adequacy of the entire episode of care. Where the judgment is of inadequate care, the specific deficiencies upon which that conclusion is based are listed.

The criteria oriented approach was used to analyze the quality of care provided by two service units. The medication maintenance–resocialization program was selected on the basis of an overall utilization profile demonstrating a bias favoring whites; the inpatient unit, because of a utilization bias favoring nonwhites. Fourteen cases were selected at random from among all patients discharged from each

Figure 3–1. An Example of Prescriptive Criteria Governing the Use
of Psychotropic Medications

---

1. Does the chart indicate the following:
   a. names of medication(s)
   b. doseages
   c. side effects or absence thereof
   d. efficacy or absence thereof

2. If medication was prescribed and adequately recorded, was it:
   a. a minor tranquilizer?

      (1) if YES, was the diagnostic number 291, 300–307, 309.13 or 316?
   b. a major tranquilizer?

      (1) if YES was the diagnostic number 290–298?
   c. an antidepressant?

      (1) If YES, was the diagnostic number 296.0, 296.2, 296.34, 298, 300.4?

3. Was a single generic variety of antidepressant given to the patient for more
   than eight months?

   (1) If YES, chart should be subject to review.

4. Has the patient received the same medication for longer than three months?

   If YES, do the total daily doseages prescribed exceed:

Valium	20 mg	Haldol	15 mg
Librium	40 mg	Navane	20 mg
Miltown	1200 mg	Thorazine	400 mg
		Mellaril	400 mg
Elavil	150 mg	Trilafon	32 mg
Tofranil	200 mg	Stelazine	30 mg
		Prolixin	10 mg

   If YES, chart should be subject to review.

5. Has the patient received the following medication in total daily dosages not
   exceeding those indicated for a period of more than six months?

Valium	5 mg		
Librium	10 mg	Thorazine	50 mg
Miltown	400 mg	Melleril	50 mg
Elavil	50 mg		
Tofranil	50 mg		

   If YES, chart should be subject to review.

unit during the preceding twelve months. Each patient so selected was then matched with a patient discharged from the same unit of different ethnicity, with age, sex, and diagnosis controlled. The results of the analysis are presented in Table 3—4.

Of the 22 issues raised in relation to the service provided by the unit where an ethnic differential favoring nonwhites existed, none pertained to the question of appropriateness. In all instances, hospitalization was felt to be justified by and consistent with the presenting problem. Six issues involving a total of three patients were raised in relation to the care provided the white patients. The clinician reviewers concurred in three instances, but made a global judgment of inadequate care in only one case. Of the five cases involving nonwhites where deviations from the criteria were noted, sixteen issues related to the process of care were raised. In eight of these instances, the clinician reviewer concurred that it indeed represented a deviation but again found only one overall episode of care to be inadequate.

A total of 28 issues involving ten cases were raised in relation to the service rendered by the unit where an ethnic differential favoring whites was noted. Of the sixteen issues raised relating to the care provided whites, clinician reviewers concurred in seven instances and judged overall care to be inadequate in two cases. Clinician reviewers concurred with issues raised in seven out of twelve instances, involving four nonwhite patients. Judgments of overall inadequacy of the treatment episode were made in three instances.

In the five instances where care was found to be inadequate, the comments of the clinical reviewers reflected a uniform opinion that the intensity of involvement provided by the program was insufficient, given the character of pathology exhibited by the patients. Comments focused upon the inappropriateness of the treatment disposition. The medication maintenance—resocialization program was felt to be an inadequate recourse in those instances where stabilization of psychosocial functioning had not been achieved.

While the sample size for this analysis was small, ethnicity does not emerge as a major predictor of the quality of services rendered. Further, there does not appear to be a relationship between the existence of ethnic differentials in patterns of care and judgments concerning how adequately providers render care to ethnic groups. It would seem that a degree of caution is in order, prior to making global pronouncements on the quality of a service or service enterprise on the basis solely of utilization data, or the analysis of patterns of care.

Table 3—4.   Ethnic Differentials in Judgments of Service Quality

	Inpatient		Medication Maintenance/ Resocialization	
	White	Nonwhite	White	Nonwhite
Cases where issues were raised by nonclinician reviewers	3	6	6	4
Types of Issues Raised				
Appropriateness of care	0 (0)	0 (0)	4 (3)	2 (2)
Adequacy of care				
Diagnosis	1 (0)	2 (1)	3 (3)	3 (2)
Treatment planning/process	4 (2)	9 (4)	4 (0)	5 (1)
Discharge planning/process	1 (1)	5 (3)	5 (2)	2 (2)
Total of Issues Raised	6 (3)	16 (8)	16 (7)	12 (7)
Episodes of care judged inadequate by clinician reviewers	1	1	2	3

( ) indicates number of instances where clinician reviewer concurred with clinical issue raised.

STUDY 5: ETHNICITY AND THE OUTCOME
OF CARE

Of course, my pronouncement suffers from not taking into account whether ethnic differentials in patterns of care tend to deprive people of the potential benefit derived from the receipt of treatment. Let me briefly describe a multidimensional outcome study that was undertaken in order to address this question.

The service assayed was one demonstrating an ethnic bias in the pattern of care favoring whites. The sample was derived from a cohort of patients randomly selected for participation in a larger study of outpatient decision making. It was composed of 34 ethnic pairs matched on age, sex, and diagnosis. Outcome measures included change in symptom discomfort and social functioning, re-entry into treatment, and satisfaction with treatment. The former involved a comparison of scale scores obtained upon admission and six months post-discharge. The instruments used were the Inventory of Psychic and Somatic Complaints and the Katz Social Adjustment Scales [9, 10]. Six major analytic domains were included in the analysis: sociodemography, symptomatology, social role performance, treatment career, treatment attitudes—motivation, and treatment outcome. The results are summarized in Figure 3—2.

For our purposes, discussion will be limited to treatment outcome. No significant association between ethnicity and outcome was noted in relation to satisfaction with treatment, re-entry into treatment, change in satisfaction with social role performance, or change in satisfaction with leisure time activities. Greater amelioration of symptom discomfort and a higher level of both social role performance and involvement in leisure time activities were reported by whites six months post-discharge. In this instance, it would appear that the bias in patterns of care favoring whites is associated with their deriving greater benefit from the receipt of services. Alternatively, the existence of a negative bias in relation to patterns of care does not necessarily imply that a particular population is being deprived of benefit.

IMPLICATIONS

As I noted at the beginning of the presentation, my intent is more cautionary than definitive. At times, the scope of inquiry has been limited by available data. It was not possible to survey the quality of care provided by each service element. The brief sortie into outcome analysis was limited to a single service. There was no opportunity to

Figure 3—2. Summary of the Results of an Outcome Study Involving 34 Ethnic Pairs Matched on Age, Sex, and Diagnosis

---

I. Sociodemographic

Marital Status
Religion**
Level of Education***
Employment Status
Income

II. Symptomatology

Level of Symptom Discomfort (Self Report)
Level of Symptom Discomfort (Significant Other)
Severity of Pathology (Clinician)

III. Social Role Performance

Overall Role Performance
Satisfaction with Role Performance
Level of Participation in Leisure Time Activities
Satisfaction with Participation in Leisure Time Activities
Overall Assessment of Social Maladaptation (Clinician)

IV. Treatment Career

Previous Hospitalization
Previous Outpatient Therapy
Previous Medications
Point of Entry
Referral Source
Treatment Modality
Length of Treatment
Frequency of Contact
Mode of Termination

V. Treatment Attitudes/Motivation

Expectations
Positive Regard
Discomfort
Negative Regard
Mutuality
Empathy
Satisfaction

VI. Treatment Outcome

Reentry into Treatment Within 6 months
Change in Symptom Discomfort (Self Report)***********************

Figure 3–2. continued

VI. Treatment Outcome *(cont'd.)*

Change in Social Role Performance*********************************
Change in Satisfaction with Social Role Performance
Change in Level of Leisure Time Activities***************************
Change in Satisfaction with Leisure Time Activities

---

compare these results with the outcome of treatment on a unit where ethnic differentials in the pattern of care took on another form. Additionally, the analyses must contend with the traditional dilemmas associated with research in the natural setting.

Having offered my apoligia, I would like to comment on certain implications of the results. Clearly, it should be difficult to assume that either the quality of service or the benefit derived from care are necessary corollaries of accessibility and availability. Similarly, generalizations concerning the excellence of a service enterprise made solely on the basis of data obtained from utilization studies or analyses of patterns of care should be suspect as they tend to oversimplify what would appear to be an extremely complex phenomenon. The degree of complexity is apparent in the results generated by the analytic sequence used to explore the relationship between ethnicity and the delivery of mental health services.

A study of the need-demand continuum revealed a high degree of concordance between ethnicity, the need for care, and the demand for service. The existence of concordance, however, was not associated with greater access to the full array of services offered by the institution. Indeed, ethnic differentials in patterns of care did not invariably favor nonwhite patients. On the other hand, a negative bias in relation to patterns of care did not influence the quality of care received by individuals or necessarily imply that a particular population subgroup was being deprived of benefit.

CONCLUSIONS

Since the topic of this conference is "A Critical Appraisal of Community Psychiatry," let me conclude by offering a set of generalizations concerning the organization and delivery of mental health services. These generalizations are based upon data from the present inquiry, as well as earlier studies of the need-demand continuum which Jerome Myers, Jerzy Henisz, and I conducted [11–15].

1. While the community has a reservoir of potential cases far in excess of the number of patients accommodated by mental health service systems, it is possible to structure such systems so as to achieve a high degree of concordance between the need for care and demand for service.

2. Broad ecologic factors can be identified that are associated with differential utilization of formal mental health service system.

3. These same factors tend to influence interactions with other elements of the human service matrix, suggesting the importance of viewing the mental health service system, as a component of a larger system of social welfare and health services.

4. The importance of system connectedness becomes all the more relevant when one considers the finding that the actual demand for mental health services is more strongly influenced by factors associated with disadvantaged social status and social isolation, than by psychological impairment.

5. The importance of disadvantaged social status and social isolation, as predictors of patienthood, argues for the presence of an array of services capable of dealing with anomie as well as symptomic individuals.

6. While the responsiveness of a mental health service system can be enhanced through clearly assigning a program service responsibility for a defined geographic area, this alone will not guarantee access to care for certain categorical populations-at-risk, i.e., substance abusers or the chronically psychotic, nor insure ecologic parity in the utilization of discrete service elements.

7. The absence of ecologic parity as reflected by biases in patterns of care, however, should not be equated with the inequitable distribution of service, the rendering of care that is of inferior quality, or the denial of benefit to population subgroups.

An Evaluation of Mental Health Services

R.B. Ellsworth

The discussion at this conference indicated that there were at least two important goals in setting up the community mental health center program for this country. One was the need to provide adequate mental health services to citizens regardless of their ability to pay. The second was to make these services available in the person's community rather than at distant mental hospitals.

By 1958, substantial evidence had accumulated indicating that socioeconomic class was strongly related to the type of mental health services that people received. Lower socioeconomic class (SEC) people were more often hospitalized than higher SEC people [10]. Even when hospitalized, higher SEC people more often received psychotherapy while lower SEC people more often received the organic therapies [15]. President Kennedy's Mental Health–Retardation Centers Act in the early 1960s was designed, in large part, to provide adequate alternatives to hospital treatment for all citizens.

A THREE-PART QUESTION

How well have the community mental health centers met the challenge of providing effective services at the local level to citizens regardless of their ability to pay? This question breaks down into three parts. First, are lower SEC people still treated more often in mental hospitals rather than in community settings? Second, are mental health services effective, as measured by pre- and post-treatment changes in adjustment and role functioning? And third, is treatment in community clinics more or less effective than treatment in mental hospitals, and for whom?

The data here come from ratings of pre- and post-treatment adjustment and role functioning of clinic clients and hospitalized patients.

Patients and clients entering several hospitals and clinics were asked to name a significant other (usually a relative) who knew them well, and to give informed consent for that significant other to rate their pre- and post-treatment community behavior and adjustment. The significant other was sent a PARS Community Adjustment Scale measuring various Personal Adjustment and Role Skill factors [4] at the beginning of treatment and again on followup. For clinic clients, followup occurred approximately 90 days after intake. For hospitalized patients, followup occurred about 90 days after release.

The analysis was based on a sample of 962 pre-treatment, and 823 post-treatment PARS Scale ratings. Followup Pars Scales were not obtained from 139 significant others who had cooperated in providing pre-treatment ratings. The average number of clinic visits was 7.3 for females and 7.9 for males. Female patients were hospitalized an average of 33 days, while male patients were hospitalized 29 days.

Results

1. Factors Related to Selection of Treatment Setting. The first question examined was whether or not socioeconomic factors played an important role in determining who received treatment in mental hospitals versus community clinics. Table 3–5 presents the pre-treatment differences between clinic and hospital treated females on a number of background and adjustment variables. The most important characteristic of clinic treated women, in contrast to hospital treated patients, was diagnosis with clinic female clients more often diagnosed as nonpsychotic and hospitalized patients most often diagnosed as psychotic.

Next in importance was the severity of pre-treatment symptoms and difficulties in role functioning. Hospitalized females showed more Confusion and Anxiety-Depression than their clinic counterparts. Also, hospitalized women were less able to function in Household Management skills and were less often involved in Outside Social activities. Having children in the home and being married was also important in differentiating between those who received treatment in clinics rather than hospitals. With respect to socioeconomic variables, income did not differentiate between women treated in clinics versus hospitals, but education did to some extent, with better educated women more often seen in clinics.

For men, the most important differences between clinic and hospital treatment were accounted for primarily by diagnosis, symptom severity, and marital status rather than socioeconomic factors. As seen in Table 3–6, clinic treated men were more often diagnosed as

Table 3–5. Initial PARS and Background Differences Between Female Clinic Clients and Hospitalized Patients

		Pretreatment PARS Means		F Ratio of Mean Differences
		Clinic N=269	Hospital N=284	
PARS Scores (Female)				
(A)	Interpersonal Relations	12.4	11.6	5.5*
(B)	Anxiety-Depression	13.5	14.9	21.2**
(C)	Confusion	12.0	14.6	59.8**
(D)	Alcohol/Drug Use	5.2	5.7	5.3*
(E)	Household Management	15.2	12.7	39.2**
(F)	Relationship to Children	11.4	11.1	1.4
(G)	Outside Social	6.8	5.2	37.9**
(H)	Employment	4.9	4.4	4.1*
Background				
(I)	Age	32.2	35.3	7.4**
(J)	Income Code	2.5	2.5	0.0
(K)	Education Code	3.0	2.6	14.7**
		Percent		*Chi Square*
(L)	Children in home	72	49	29.0**
(M)	Currently married	78	60	20.3**
(N)	Once married	11	22	11.5**
(O)	Never married	11	18	4.9*
(P)	Spouse as rater	63	50	9.1**
(Q)	Parent as rater	15	24	7.4**
(R)	"Other" as rater	22	25	0.6
(S)	Diagnosis			
	Alcohol	4	4	0.0
	Non-Psychotic	79	30	129.9**
	Psychotic	7	64	194.4**
	Other	11	1	23.3**

*$p < .05$
**$p < .01$

nonpsychotic while hospitalized men were more often diagnosed as psychotic. Almost of equal importance to diagnosis was employment, with clinic clients more often working than hospitalized males. Hospital treated men were also rated as more Anxious, Agitated-Depressed, and Confused than their clinic treated counterparts. As with women, male clinic clients more often were married and came from homes with children, than hospitalized patients. And finally, socioeconomic status differentiated the clinic and hospital male groups to some extent in that clinic clients had higher incomes and more education than hospitalized patients.

**Table 3–6. Initial PARS and Background Differences Between Male
Clinic Clients and Hospitalized Patients**

| | | Pretreatment PARS Means | | F Ratio of Mean Differences |
		Clinic N=183	Hospital N=226	
PARS Scores (Male)				
(A)	Interpersonal Relations	12.0	11.3	3.1
(B)	Agitation-Depression	11.0	13.3	29.3**
(C)	Anxiety	9.3	11.4	47.0**
(D)	Confusion	11.5	13.6	27.7**
(E)	Alcohol/Drugs	7.8	9.8	19.6**
(F)	Relationship to Children	9.9	9.6	1.3
(G)	Outside Social	7.2	6.0	2.1
(H)	Employment	8.5	6.1	53.9**
Background				
(I)	Age	34.4	35.3	0.5
(J)	Income Code	2.8	2.2	21.4**
(K)	Education Code	2.9	2.5	13.5**
		Percent		Chi Square
(L)	Children in home	67	41	33.6**
(M)	Currently married	75	47	30.2**
(N)	Once married	6	17	10.4**
(O)	Never married	19	36	13.4**
(P)	Spouse rated	73	43	35.2**
(Q)	Parent as rater	11	27	16.0**
(R)	"Other" as rater	16	30	10.3**
(S)	Diagnosis			
	Alcohol	15	29	10.8**
	Non-Psychotic	70	28	66.6**
	Psychotic	8	40	50.7**
	Other	7	2	5.4

$*p < .05$
$**p < .01$

Although diagnosis was an important predictor of hospital versus clinic treatment for both men and women, the act of seeking admission to a psychiatric hospital has been found to result in a high probability of normal persons being diagnosed as schizophrenic [16]. Thus, a diagnosis of psychosis partly reflects the severity of symptoms, as seen in Tables 3–5 and 3–6. But, it also reflects the fact that a person who presents himself to a hospital rather than a clinic is more likely to be diagnosed as psychotic because that diagnosis is more readily used in hospital settings.

The conclusions drawn from these two tables indicate that symptom severity and role performance were the most important factors in determining who received treatment in mental hospitals rather than in community clinics. If a person was very Confused, Anxious, Agitated-Depressed, and diagnosed as psychotic, he or she was more likely to be treated in a mental hospital. In the areas of role performance, those who were not breadwinners, homemakers, spouses, or parents were also more likely to go to a mental hospital for treatment. Thus, symptom severity and role performance were the important predictors of who received treatment in mental hospitals, rather than socioeconomic status, which was less predictive of treatment setting.

2. The Effectiveness of Mental Health Services. As can be seen in Table 3–7, the largest changes in the pre- and post-treatment adjustment of females occurred in the areas of symptom severity for both clinic and hospital treated female patients. For both female groups, the changes in Confusion and Anxiety-Depression were the most significant. Interpersonal Involvement also improved for both clinic and hospital treated females. In the Role Skill areas, the changes in Household Management, Outside Social, and Parenthood Skills were most significant, while Employment scores showed no change.

The greatest improvement for males was also shown in the area of symptom severity. As seen in Table 3–8, the areas of Confusion, Anxiety, and Agitation-Depression showed the most significant changes. Interpersonal Involvement showed some improvement, but

Table 3–7. Pre-treatment and Post-treatment Adjustment Means for Hospitalized and Clinic Females

	Clinic Females			Hospitalized Females		
	Pre	Post	t value	Pre	Post	t value
Interpersonal Inv.	12.5	13.6	5.06**	11.6	13.9	8.26**
Confusion	12.1	10.2	8.18**	14.2	10.5	12.73**
Anxiety-Depression	13.6	11.1	10.08**	14.6	10.5	14.95**
Alcohol/Drug	5.2	5.0	1.99*	5.7	4.7	6.42**
Household Mgm.	15.0	15.5	2.27*	13.0	14.6	5.52**
Outside Social	6.7	7.4	3.74**	5.3	5.8	3.24**
Parenthood Skills	11.5	12.0	3.01**	11.2	12.4	4.53**
Employment	4.9	5.0	0.93	4.5	4.6	0.52

$*p < .05$ for appropriate df
$**p < .01$ for appropriate df

Table 3–8.   Pre-treatment and Post-treatment Adjustment Means
for Clinic and Hospitalized Males

	Clinic Clients			Hospitalized Males		
	Pre	Post	t value	Pre	Post	t value
1. Interpersonal Inv.	12.1	12.7	2.44*	11.7	12.8	3.65**
2. Confusion	11.6	10.1	5.40**	13.3	10.2	10.00**
3. Anxiety	9.4	7.9	5.71**	11.5	8.4	11.54**
4. Agitation-Depression	10.9	9.6	4.29**	12.9	9.5	10.4**
5. Alcohol/Drug	7.8	7.1	2.91**	10.1	7.5	7.95**
6. Outside Social	7.1	7.2	0.84	6.0	6.6	2.83**
7. Parenthood Skills	9.7	10.4	2.57*	9.7	10.8	2.95**
8. Employment	8.4	8.2	0.83	6.5	6.6	0.71

*$p < .05$ for appropriate df
**$p < .01$ for appropriate df

less than that shown by women. There was also a significant decrease in Alcohol/Drug Use, especially by hospitalized patients. And finally, the Role Skill areas of Outside Social and Employment showed little or no improvement in either clinic or hospital treated groups.

These findings are consistent with those reported elsewhere, namely, that treatment in mental health settings has a greater impact on personal adjustment and symptoms than on role skills [6]. Mental health services, therefore, are especially effective in providing relief from distressing symptoms.

3. The Comparative Effectiveness of Hospital Versus Clinic Treatment. Did patients who went to hospitals have a different outcome than those seen in community clinics? In his review of available data, Arnhoff [1] found no evidence that treatment in community settings was more effective in helping people with adjustment problems than hospital treatment. While the monetary cost for clinic treated clients may be less than that for hospital treated patients, the social cost to the family and community is often very high if patients are treated in a community setting when emotionally disturbed and poorly functioning.

One problem in answering this question of comparative effectiveness of hospital versus clinic treatment is choosing the best way of measuring improvement or treatment outcome. Change scores and post-treatment outcome scores are both highly correlated with initial adjustment [5, 12, 18]. Change scores tend to favor patients with poor pre-treatment adjustment, since such patients show more pre-post change than initially well adjusted patients. Outcome scores, on the other hand, favor initially well adjusted patients since these patients also tend to have better outcome scores. Since there were clear differences in the initial adjustment of clinic clients and hospitalized patients (as seen above in Tables 3—5 and 3—6), neither change scores nor post-treatment outcome scores could be used to answer the question of who had the best treatment outcome, clinic clients or hospital patients.

Methods for calculating post-treatment scores have been suggested by several investigators [2, 3, 11]. A frequently used approach is to remove that portion of the outcome score that is a function of the initial level of adjustment. These corrected or residual outcome scores are "base-free," in that they are not correlated with initial adjustment differences. As such, residual scores are more likely to reflect treatment effects rather than initial differences among patients.

As seen in Table 3—9, females treated in hospitals had higher residual post-treatment scores than their clinic counterparts on

Table 3—9. Adjusted Residual Outcome Scores for Clinic Clients and Hospitalized Patients

		Residual Outcome Scores		t-test Mean Difference
PARS Factor Dimensions		*Clinic N=227*	*Hospital N=249*	
(1)	*Females*			
(A)	Interpersonal Relations	−.45	.26	2.38*
(B)	Anxiety-Depression	.56	−.47	3.22**
(C)	Confusion	.49	−.26	2.46*
(D)	Alcohol/Drugs	.29	−.24	3.74**
(E)	Household Management	−.15	.07	0.70
(F)	Relationship to Children	−.21	.26	1.85
(G)	Outside Social	.30	−.36	3.04**
(H)	Employment	.12	−.11	1.10
(2)	*Males*	*N=151*	*N=196*	
(A)	Interpersonal Relations	−.28	.24	1.47
(B)	Agitation-Depression	.38	−.38	2.01*
(C)	Anxiety	.08	−.04	0.37
(D)	Confusion	.29	−.28	1.62
(E)	Alcohol/Drugs	.29	−.21	1.58
(F)	Relationship to Children	.02	−.05	0.27
(G)	Outside Social	.14	−.22	1.36
(H)	Employment	−.21	.26	1.08

*p < .05
**p < .01

Interpersonal Relations, and lower residual scores in the areas of Anxiety-Depression, Confusion, Alcohol/Drug Use, and Outside Social. Controlling for the effects of differences in initial adjustment, then, females treated in hospitals had better treatment outcomes in the Personal Adjustment areas than clinic clients. The only Role Skill area on which clinic and hospital treated females differed was Outside Social, where hospital treated females continued to function less well (lower residual outcome) than their clinic counterparts.

For males, those treated in hospitals were not clearly better adjusted on followup except in the area of Agitation-Depression. Hospital treated males tended to show lower residual psychopathology scores on followup, but the differences between patients and clients did not usually reach an acceptable level of statistical significance.

A related question was whether or not the four groups (females and males treated in hospitals and clinics) differed in treatment outcome from each other. Since the PARS Scales for males and females differ in item content, treatment outcomes for the four groups could not be compared for all areas of adjustment. There are, however, six items that sample anxiety, depression, and confusion, and are common on both male and female PARS Scales. Using these six items, maladjustment scores were obtained for all four groups, and residual outcome scores were computed.

An overall F ratio of 2.76 ($p < .05$ for 3 and 798 df) was obtained for the residual maladjustment outcome scores of the four groups, indicating that some significant outcome differences had occurred between groups. A Duncan Range test revealed that females treated in hospitals had lower residual maladjustment scores (-0.62) than either females or males treated in clinics (0.40 and 0.32 respectively). Males treated in hospitals had intermediate residual maladjustment scores (0.07) that were not statistically different from any of the other three groups. In general, then, women treated in hospitals tended to have the best treatment outcome.

The finding that women treated in hospital settings showed greater symptom reduction than women seen in clinics, is consistent with Arnhoff's [1] conclusion that there is no evidence that community-based treatment is more effective than hospital treatment. In fact, the reverse may be more accurate for women—namely, that hospital treatment reduces symptoms of psychological distress to a greater extent than community treatment. The finding of a possible sex-linked response to treatment has also been reported by Evenson [7] and Hogarty et al. [9]. In the present study, a hospital stay averaging 30 days for females can be regarded as more intensive than seven clinic visits. Thus there is some evidence that women show more improvement than men when receiving intensive treatment, including hospitalization.

Comment

The data presented in this paper suggest that the community mental health movement has met some of the goals originally envisioned, but not all of them. A much higher percentage of people are being treated in community settings now than in the 1950s. There was evidence that socioeconomic status does not now play as important a role as it apparently did in the first half of this century in determining which people went to mental hospitals for treatment and which ones were seen in community settings. The evidence presented in this paper also indicated that symptom severity and role performance were among the most important predictors of which setting a person went to for treatment.

The data presented also indicated that mental health services were more effective for some areas of adjustment and functioning than for others. There was clear evidence that more improvement occurred in the symptom and personal adjustment areas than in the role skills, a finding reported in other studies. The finding that hospital treatment was more effective in reducing symptomatology for women than clinic treatment, may surprise many of those who initially proposed that community treatment would be more effective than treatment received in mental hospitals. Not only was there no evidence that community-based treatment programs were more effective than hospital treatment, but it was found that hospital treatment was actually more effective than clinic treatment for females.

A major problem in evaluating the effectiveness of mental health services is that very few treatment settings collect any data on the treatment outcomes of their patients and clients. A great deal of increased effort is being expended on various review activities, such as peer reviews, medical audits, quality assurance committees, joint commission audits, accreditation standards, utilization reviews, external and internal audits. But this constitutes monitoring the treatment processes, not outcomes, I do not believe that process monitoring will increase program effectiveness or reduce costs. By setting standards for what staff do rather than on the effects of services rendered, we run the very real risk of stifling innovations and increasing costs rather than decreasing them.

There is no evidence that I know of to demonstrate that treatment effectiveness is improved when certain diagnostic procedures are utilized, when records are kept in prescribed ways, when certain kinds of services are made available, or when peers decide from examining records that adequate treatment was rendered. At this point almost nothing is known about which of our many activities help increase treatment effectiveness and which practices do not. And yet we operate as if we know which of our services are important for increasing treatment effectiveness.

I believe that much more of our effort should be devoted to assessing treatment outcome rather than monitoring treatment process. One reason for not assessing outcome in past years is that it has been much more difficult to measure outcome than to monitor process. But certain recent advances have been made in developing more adequate and less costly methods for measuring the impact of treatment on a client's adjustment and social functioning. Let me summarize briefly some of the recent findings regarding the measurement of outcome.

First, professionally trained staff are not necessary for assessing the pre- and post-treatment of clients. In reaching conclusions about which treatment approach was most effective, ratings from patients and their relatives typically yield the same conclusions as those based on ratings by professional staff [9, 13, 14].

The *second* recent finding is that ratings of adjustment in the treatment setting do not correlate with adjustment ratings in the community setting [5, 6]. Therefore, adequate program evaluation should be based on ratings of functioning in the community setting.

The *third* recent finding is that mental health services affect different areas of adjustment and functioning in different ways [8]. As already seen, patients and clients show clear pre–post-treatment improvement in such areas as anxiety, depression, confusion, etc. Most of the improvement in these areas tends to be maintained over time following treatment. While there is initial improvement in the area of alcohol abuse, improvement in this area is generally not maintained over time. Employment, on the other hand, is generally lower immediately following residential treatment, but tends to rise over time to the level of pre-treatment employment. These findings by Fontana [8] indicate that one should use multidimensional scales in assessing outcome, for different areas of adjustment and functioning are affected differently by mental health services.

A *fourth* conclusion that I have reached is that program effectiveness can be assessed routinely without the use of control groups or random assignment to treatments. Most treatment agencies have not been able to justify withholding treatment or assigning clients randomly in order to evaluate program effectiveness. A recent innovation that I feel will be of great help in program evaluation is the development of "change norms" [5]. These norms indicate how much change typically occurs in patients treated in hospitals, as well as with clients treated in clinics.

With these kinds of change norms available, a clinic or hospital can determine whether their patients or clients change more or less, than similar patients or clients treated in other settings. If a particular treatment approach or agency obtained more change than was found for similar clients in other programs, then a more controlled comparison outcome study could be planned. In this way, the special effort required for such comparison studies would be reserved only when it seemed that a particular program was unusually effective or ineffective.

IN SUMMARY

Recent developments have shown that program evaluation does not require the expense of professionally trained raters. Questionnaires with adequate psychometric properties have been developed for use by clients and their relatives for assessing pre–post-treatment changes [17]. Second, evaluation of treatment outcome should be based on ratings of community adjustment and functioning rather than ratings made in the treatment setting. Community-based ratings can be obtained inexpensively by mail from clients and their significant others. Third, one needs to assess outcome with scales that measure various aspects of both personal adjustment and role functioning. This is necessary because different areas of adjustment and functioning are affected differently by mental health services. And fourth, the assessment of program effectiveness does not require the routine use of control groups nor random assignment to treatments. Controlled studies are necessary only when the routine monitoring of program effectiveness suggests that a particular program is unusually effective or ineffective.

It seems to me that the recent emphasis on monitoring treatment process is not likely to improve effectiveness nor to reduce costs, but could well have the opposite effects. Much more attention needs to be paid to evaluating pre–post-treatment changes of clients and patients in mental health programs. Although there is no guarantee at this time that evaluating outcomes will immediately increase program effectiveness, I believe it will focus attention on a much more important area than process monitoring. If attention and effort were directed more to outcome evaluation, and less to process monitoring, people would be much more likely to find ways of increasing program effectiveness. As things stand now, no mental health agency knows how effective its services are compared to other agencies.

Discussant I: Assessing the Development of Community Psychiatry

Thomas J. Kiresuk
Sander Lund

The purpose of this paper is to examine and expand upon some of the issues raised by Mosher and Tischler regarding the development and current status of the community psychiatry movement. In the course of this undertaking, relevant findings will be outlined from a large scale mental health evaluation study sponsored in Hennepin County, Minnesota by the National Institute of Mental Health, and an attempt will be made to link what has been presented to the larger shaping issues of this conference.

Mosher's paper on the politicization of policy seems to exclude medical and academic settings. Political maneuvering is not the exclusive province of government, and it seems essential that the political aspects of research and practice in mental health also receive special study. The allocation of resources in professional settings is a function of more than objective fact, and other sources of influence must be understood if they are to be dealt with.

One essential problem in the community mental health system may relate to the issue referred to by Lynn and Salasin (1974) in *Evaluation* magazine as "human services shortfall," or the explicit promising of human services unjustified by either current knowledge or current resources. The raising of unmeetable expectations can easily lead to anger, frustration, and cynicism. If we did "promise a rose garden," prior declaration of policy expectations and outcomes might have alerted us to the magnitude of our optimism, or at least might have had a mitigating effect upon the popular disenchantment engendered by our failure to meet all needs.

Mosher's emphasis on the importance of the total political, social, and regulatory context within which community psychiatry has developed is absolutely correct. Mental health programs do not operate in a vacuum, and, in fact, the sociopolitical environment surrounding and supporting an organization is the ultimate reference point for total evaluation systems. It is ironic that many of us who assumed that we shared a common value system with the "community" have discovered that the notions of professionals represent only another minority opinion.

One source of dissonance among the competing value systems relates to medical domination of the mental health enterprise, and it may be concluded that the application of the "medical model" to mental health activities commits the error of many another discipline, that of confounding a theory of health and illness with a preference for administrative authority. Fortunately, these two issues are being neatly disentangled by administrators and policy makers.

Mosher attributes the low appreciation of evaluation in the community psychiatry movement to a lack of backing by law, prestige, and power. While this contention seems largely true, it should also be pointed out that the evaluation and research process in mental health has often been uniquely characterized by irrelevance: irrelevance to law, irrelevance to clinicians, irrelevance to consumers and community, irrelevance, in fact, to just about everything but research itself. Evaluation must, like the larger field of mental health, recognize the importance of its interdependent relationship with the surrounding culture. In order to insure that the results of their endeavors are meaningful and useful, evaluators must forge strong links between their discipline and value systems of its community of users.

Mosher also presumes that a program must hold still to be evaluated. Until recently there would have been widespread agreement with this position; however, in the last few years the concept of formative evaluation has come to prominence. Distinguished by Scrivens (1967) from "summative evaluation," which is a final, one-shot summation of a program's worth, "formative evaluation" is the periodic review and monitoring of a program to obtain "knowledge of results" feedback to improve performance. Formative evaluation attempts to maximize utilization of evaluation information, and, as Mosher notes (indeed as all of the papers presented seem to emphasize), one of the major shortcomings of the mental health field seems to be a failure to appropriately utilize derived knowledge.

Failure to obtain reasonable benefit from the results of research and evaluation is at least as important at the interprogram as at the intraprogram level. A significant (but discouraging) finding of a recent National Institute of Mental Health survey was that even exemplary innovations were discontinued by mental health programs once initial federal support was discontinued. Poor knowledge transfer and lack of incentive for innovation can be subsumed under the larger topic of diffusion and utilization of knowledge. The work of Davis (1973), Rogers (1962), Zaltman (1973), Glaser (1973), and others relates to a literature of over 20,000 citations on this topic. Research is currently underway to isolate the essential components of successful knowledge transfer, and to use this information as a springboard for the development of a detailed and systematic technology of planned change.

One explanation for the lack of public interest noted by Mosher in community psychiatry may be that the values of the public were not formally consulted in the first place. Professional and political values tend to be well represented in community mental health, but the viewpoints of the consumer, and of the general public, remain in the province of something like cultural anthropology. Ralph Nader (Chu and Trotter, 1973) has already turned a somewhat critical eye toward the mental health establishment, and unless a mechanism is established to incorporate outside feedback into the direction of the movement, community psychiatry may become an advisarial rather than a cooperative venture. As Mosher notes, room must be made for diversity, and creativity and legitimate deviance must be encouraged. This view point, however, constitutes only one more value system— one of many that must be accommodated.

Tischler's paper seems to represent an attempt to apply a framework of scientific justification, in a humane and personal way, to the ultimate needs of mental health. His concern for perceived and evaluated need is a means to approach the problem of the ultimate relevance of community psychiatry, a point alluded to by Mr. Kittay, when he suggested that business criteria might be applied to our specialty to help determine where current values rest: resource allocation being an immediate indicator of value commitment. However, Tischler's formulation is careful to leave a buffer zone for the development of subsystems that are selective and may operate counter to social policy objectives. This strikes a harmonic with the results of the work in Hennepin County and with Mosher's concern for the conservation of "legitimate deviance."

Tischler also shows a respect for audit mechanisms that monitor the congruence between professional activities and the larger values of the mental health services delivery system, but he cautions that utilization review procedures alone can be misleading with regard to a program's worth. This concern is consistent with results from a Hennepin County study which related to treatment dropouts. Despite the fact that they are under utilizing available resources, they seem to be doing just fine.

Tischler seems to advocate opening the community psychiatry

field to multiple value systems, and reasons that mere "effectiveness" is not the only reason for insuring equal accessibility and availability of services (minorities have the same right to spend money on ineffective treatment, placebo effects, and spontaneous remissions that whites have). If the question of where minorities should sit in a bus were evaluated only from the perspective of efficient and effective transportation, without reference to the supporting cultural values, an objective evaluation would probably conclude that discriminatory seating constitutes no significant difference from free choice. By relating the focus of community psychiatry to factors beyond immediate psychological impairment, Tischler points to evaluation grounded in concepts that transcend traditional concepts of efficacy in relieving client distress.

A New Method Proposed

The balance of this paper is intended to propose a method that could shape and lead mental health programs toward meeting the needs of their multiple constituencies in a manner amenable to objective assessment and rational control. Such a method would incorporate past and current evaluation findings; would be responsive to changes in goals; would include and be sensitive to political, social, philosophic, and administrative realities; and would conform to the various auditing procedures required by Medicaid, Medicare, hospital accreditation boards, professional standards review organizations, and the problem oriented medical records procedure. The method would also (hopefully) answer basic business questions related to effectiveness and efficiency; would detect malfunctions and facilitative effects within the service system; and would relate to the realities of stimulating change.

The prototype for the proposed method was developed at Hennepin County Mental Health Service, Minneapolis, through a grant from the National Institute of Mental Health. After an evaluation device to assess attainment of individualized client goals had been implemented, a prominent management consultant commented that what had been accomplished was irrelevant to the larger context of a mental health program's enterprise. As clinicians and administrators, staff had not recognized that there is such a thing as a "theory of an organization" comparable to a theory in science, with postulates, a priories, and a special language that reflects the value system of the organization and the socioculture context within which it operates.

The nature of this value system is quite easy to determine and incorporate into a total evaluation system. It is contained in the laws, the statutes, the policies, and the records of professional decision making. Since many of these mandates and activities have direct influence on client outcomes, one aspect of the proposed new system is an attempt to shift the focus of evaluation measurement from that of the psychometric expert to that of mental health clinicians and administrators. A second aspect is an attempt to measure traits and attributes according to outcome estimates based upon realistic, individualized treatment prognoses.

The new method is called "goal attainment scaling," and was originally described in an article by Kiresuk and Sherman (1968). An example of how the technique can be used to develop a set of client specific treatment criteria is presented in Figure 3–3. The grid shaped form itself is called a "goal attainment followup guide," and its content was determined at the time of intake for a particular client of Hennepin County Crisis Intervention Center. The staff member responsible for the client, with the input of the client in some cases, determined five problem areas were relevant to that treatment episode: "Education," "Drug Use," "Manipulation," "Suicide," and "Dependency."

Once these problem areas had been identified, an estimate was made for each regarding where the client would be at followup (three months, in this instance, from the outset of treatment), given the fact that treatment had occurred. Bracketing this estimate, or prognosis, is a scale of related outcomes, ranging from "Best Anticipated Success" to "Most Unfavorable Outcome Thought Likely." This range of possible outcomes is tailored to the client so that it constitutes an estimated normal curve of probabilities around the most likely, or "Expected Level of Treatment Success." The numbers in the title cell above each scale indicate the weight, or relative importance, of that problem area. The asterisks indicate the cell that best described the client's status at the time of intake; the checkmarks indicate the cell that best described the client's status at the time of followup.

From the ratings at the time of followup a summary goal attainment score may be calculated. Such a statistic is a general indicator of the degree to which treatment expectations have been met. The formula for calculating a goal attainment score is contained in an insert in Figure 3–4. In substance, the product of the formula is an average of attainment on all scales, adjusted for the weights of the scales, the number of scales, and the intercorrelation among the scales. Goal attainment scores generated in the same setting, and through a uniform set of procedures, typically approximate a normal distribution, with a mean of about 50.00 and a standard deviation of about 10.00. In goal attainment scaling, a score of 50.00 indicates

Figure 3−3. Sample Clinical Guide: Crisis Intervention Center

Level at Intake: $\checkmark$

Level at Follow-up: *

GOAL ATTAINMENT FOLLOW-UP GUIDE

Check whether or not the scale has been mutually negotiated between patient and CIC interviewer. SCALE ATTAINMENT LEVELS	SCALE HEADINGS AND SCALE WEIGHTS	
	Yes X No ___ SCALE 1: Education (w₁=20)	Yes ___ No X SCALE 2: Suicide (w₂=30)
a. most unfavorable treatment outcome (-2) thought likely	Patient has made no attempt to enroll in high school. $\checkmark$	Patient has committed suicide.
b. less than expected success (-1) with treatment	Patient has enrolled in high school, but at time of follow-up has dropped out.	Patient has acted on at least one suicidal impulse since her first contact with the CIC, but has not succeeded. $\checkmark$
c. expected level of treatment (0) success	Patient has enrolled, and is in school at follow-up, but is attending class sporadically (misses an average of more than a third of her classes during a week).	Patient reports she has had at least four suicidal impulses since her first contact with the CIC but has not acted on any of them.
d. more than expected success (+1) with treatment	Patient has enrolled, is in school at follow-up, and is attending classes consistently, but has no vocational goals. *	*
e. best anticipated success (+2) with treatment	Patient has enrolled, is in school at follow-up, is attending classes consistently, and has some vocational goal.	Patient reports she has had no suicidal impulses since her first contact with the CIC.

where $w_1=20$ and $w_2=30$.

Figure 3−3. continued

Level at Intake:		29.4
Goal Attainment Score		
(Level at Follow-up):		62.2
Goal Attainment Change		
Score:		+32.8

SCALE HEADINGS AND SCALE WEIGHTS (cont'd.)

Yes ___ No _X_   Yes _X_ No ___   Yes _X_ No ___

SCALE 3: Manipulation	SCALE 4: Drug Abuse	SCALE 5: Dependency on CIC
(w₃=25)	(w₄=30)	(w₅=10)
Patient makes rounds of community service agencies demanding medication, and refuses other forms of treatment ✓	Patient reports addiction to "hard narcotics" (heroin, morphine).	Patient has contacted CIC by telephone or in person at least seven times since his first visit.
Patient no longer visits CIC with demands for medication but continues with other community agencies and still refuses other forms of treatment.	Patient has used "hard narcotics," but is not addicted, and/or uses hallucinogens (LSD, Pot) more than four times a month. ✓	Patient has contacted CIC 5-6 times since intake. ✓
Patient no longer attempts to manipulate for drugs at community service agencies, but will not accept another form of treatment.	Patient has not used "hard narcotics" during follow-up period, and uses hallucinogens between 1-4 times a month. *	Patient has contacted CIC 3-4 times since intake.
Patient accepts non-medication treatment at some community agency. *	Patient uses hallucinogens less than once a month.	
Patient accepts non-medication treatment, and by own report shows signs of improvement.	At time of follow-up, patient is not using any illegal drugs.	Patient has not contacted CIC since intake. *

Figure 3−4.   Formulas for Calculating Goal Attainment Score and Distribution of Goal Attainment Scores from Hennepin County Mental Health Center

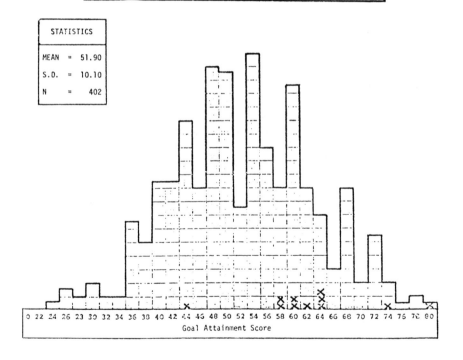

Original Goal Attainment Score formula:

$$T_j = 50 + \frac{10\Sigma w_i x_i}{\sqrt{(1-\rho)\Sigma w_i^2 + \rho(\Sigma w_i)^2}}$$

where it is recommended that ρ be taken as about .30.

Modified Goal Attainment formula:

$$T' = 50 + \frac{\Sigma w_j(T_j-50)}{\sqrt{(1-\rho)\Sigma w_j^2 + \rho(\Sigma w_j)^2}}$$

where it may be necessary to select a value for ρ commensurate with the intercorrelations of the sub-objective scores, T_j

STATISTICS

MEAN = 51.90

S.D. = 10.10

N   = 402

Goal Attainment Score

that, on the average, all treatment expectations have been exactly attained; a score of more than 50.00 indicates that expectations have been exceeded; a score of less than 50.00 indicates that outcome has fallen short of expectations.

Figure 3–4 shows the distribution of goal attainment scores for the first 402 clients followed up at Hennepin County Mental Health Service. Both clients randomly and nonrandomly assigned to treatment are included in the distribution. The little x's on the abscissa of the graph indicate the scores of clients assigned to one therapist, a format which allows the clinician receiving feedback to compare individual performance with that of the organization's total community of therapists. Feedback of goal attainment scores to therapists at the Mental Health Service was initiated only after a large number of followups had been completed, and a comparison of clinicians' scores before feedback with those after feedback revealed a statistically significant positive change in goal attainment score (Walker and Baxter, 1972).

After nearly 700 clients have been followed up, the first phase of the goal attainment scaling evaluation of Hennepin County Mental Health Service was terminated, and a systematic analysis of the data begun. The results of this analysis show significant differences in outcome score between individual therapists and within disciplines (psychiatry, clinical psychology, social work, psychiatric nursing), but no differences among disciplines or among treatment modes (individual psychotherapy, group therapy, day hospital treatment, medications).

Currently, the Mental Health Service maintains a comprehensive formative evaluation system founded in goal attainment scaling, and featuring aspects of (1) organizational level management by objectives, (2) process evaluation through an automated management information system, and (3) client outcome evaluation according to attainment of individualized treatment goals. In this system, clinical goals are negotiated with the client by an intake worker, and the case is then assigned (randomly, whenever possible) to an independent therapist.

To insure that the content of the followup guide is not capricious or irrelevant, all scales are audited by clinical staff to determine whether they are relevant and realistic and whether the weights were appropriate. This is a potential access point for "significant others," such as consumer advocates, patient representatives, and professional organizations. Followup assessment of goal attainment occurs at a time agreed upon by intake worker and client, typically two to six months after treatment begins, and involves a personal interview between client and therapist. As an accountability check, every tenth followup is verified by an independent interviewer.

Figure 3–5 demonstrates that we are not achieving our goals at the expense of our patients, but that there is a direct and positive association between goal attainment score and client estimation of outcome. In addition, multiple reliability studies have been undertaken, and show that specialists are not required either to build scales or to score them. Sherman (1975) maintains that if you grant the assumption that mental health workers are competent to select relevant goals and scale accurate prognoses, the only major technical question related to goal attainment scaling is the reliability of outcome scoring.

Using components of variance, Sherman, Baxter and Audette (1974) have been able to show that between 50 and 65 percent of the variation in goal attainment scores is associated with actual client change. Although difficult to compare with measures having fixed or standard content, additional reliability measures analagous to test retest (.83) and scorer agreement (.66 to .81) suggest that there is enough stability in the goal attainment score to permit its use as a general indicator of effectiveness of community mental health treatment.

Probably the most important finding to date is that patients themselves can select and scale meaningful treatment goals. A self-administering form of goal attainment scaling has been developed by Garwick (1973) and was first tested at the Hennepin County Day Hospital Program. The initial intention of the study was to determine if clients could indeed perform the relatively complex task of select-

Figure 3–5. Goal Attainment Score as a Function of Consumer Satisfaction, Item #7: "How Do You Feel Now as Compared to When You First Came for Services?"

Response	N	Mean Goal Attainment Score	Standard Deviation	Standard Error of Mean
Much Worse	6	39.68	13.72	5.60
Worse	19	36.43	9.58	2.20
Same	74	45.18	8.12	.94
Better	331	50.46	10.30	.57
Much Better	263	57.06	10.67	.66
Total	693	51.92	11.32	.43

F value from ANOVA = 39.24 ($p < .01$)

ing goals and scaling possible outcomes. Presuming patients possessed this capacity, a second objective of the study was to assess the congruency between client goals and clinician goals.

To attain the second objective, goal attainment followup guides were constructed by staff for all patients, while half the patients were randomly selected to also scale their own goals. A serendipitous finding of this study was that clients who scaled their own goals did significantly better on the criteria established by staff, than did the clients who did not use goal attainment scaling (Jones and Garwick, 1973) (see Figure 3–6). This effect, which seems to provide support for the practice of allowing clients significant input in determining the course of their treatment, has been verified by Smith (1976) and LaFerriere and Calysn (1975).

Constructive Program Change

The final point of this paper relates not to goal attainment scaling, but rather to the broader topic of the stimulation and facilitation of constructive program change in mental health organizations. Years of experience in attempting to install goal attainment scaling in mental health settings has verified the conclusion reached earlier by formal students of change: that the likelihood of enduring constructive change in a system is a function of more than the merits of the particular innovation involved; the receptivity of the system itself must also be considered.

Research is currently underway in Hennepin County based upon the "A VICTORY" model of organizational readiness to innovate

Figure 3–6. Comparative Clinician-Constructed Goal Attainment Scores for Clients Randomly Allocated to Groups Using and Not Using the "Guide to Goals" Format to Scale Their Own Treatment Goals

	N	*Mean*	*S.D.*
Group 1: Used "Guide to Goals" Format.	7	71.2	6.57
Group 2: Did Not Use "Guide to Goals" Format.	7	59.2	9.88
Totals	14	65.2	—

Standard Error (difference, $\bar{X}_1 - \bar{X}_2$) $= 4.48$ ($df = 12$)

$t_{(12)} = 2.68$ ($p < .05$)

(Davis and Salasin, 1976). This model postulates that eight factors are crucial in the success or failure of a particular innovation: the Ability of the organization to change, the Values of the organization, the quality of Information regarding the change, the Circumstances attendant to the change, the Timing of the change with other events, the Obligation of the organization to change, the Resistances to the change, and the potential Yield of the change. Ultimately, the predictive accuracy of this model will be determined in regard to aspects of the course of organizational change, and technical assistance strategies will be tailored to particular constellations of the eight factors.

An important aspect of the appraisal of community psychiatry is measurement: not only of the effectiveness of direct services, but also of the progress of the movement as a whole. Without prior specifications of intentions and expectations, a meaningful set of performance criteria will be lacking to future conferences and a similar difficulty will be faced in assessing progress and planning activities. A protean measurement device such as goal attainment scaling seems uniquely suited to the task of generating such criteria.

One of the signal advantages of goal attainment measurement devices is that they allow multiple input in the selection and scaling of goals. An evolving movement such as community psychiatry must address many audiences and mediate among many viewpoints. The open-ended aspect of goal attainment measurement devices provides an opportunity to encompass and integrate a multitude of value systems. In addition, because they provide for individualized problem definition, such devices allow subsystems of the main enterprise to formulate goals of their own. Formative social movements seem to grow best from pluralistic bases, and, as Mosher suggests, some value systems cannot and should not be buried in the whole. Presuming agreement on a common mission, one means to encourage healthy diversity is to allow those with different, even conflicting expectations to scale their goals using the goal attainment format. Public dissemination of such goals tends to stimulate communication and facilitative competition at the same time that it provides an indication as to the overall status of the field.

Even setting aside the related technical issues of the Bayesian approach to research, sound interpretation of scientific findings requires reference to nonscientific value judgments. Is it, for example, "good" that state hospital censuses have been significantly reduced? Is the recidivism rate for schizophrenics "too high" or "about what we should expect" or "good enough to leave alone" from the point of view of the dedication of research resources? What should we have expected from the community mental health movement? Using goal attainment scaling, the answers to such questions would be rephrased into, "is the achievement indicated by a goal attainment score of 50.00 and its related specific, prior expectations sufficient, mediocre, or bordering on the unethical?"

It is no particular secret that at its worst, evaluation is aversive, and at its best is probably less interesting than many other professional activities. Yet without "knowledge of results" feedback we lack, both as a movement and as individual practitioners, a reliable guide for the course of future development. Community psychiatry is a progressive and vital force, and can be proud of its many significant accomplishments. Nonetheless, subsequent achievement may well depend upon the degree to which we can agree upon and publically disseminate our real standards of success. Accountability can be more than a political shibboleth, and more than a bureaucratic tangle of paperwork. It can be our link with the larger culture and our vehicle for learning from the past.

Discussant II: The Quality of Delivery of Mental Health Services to the Community

Ira Glick

My task, is to do two things. First, to discuss the paper of Dr. Tischler. Second, to present our own work as it related to evaluation and hopefully to integrate our data with those of Dr. Ellsworth.

My central thesis is that the community mental health system is a major achievement and a major step forward, but that it still leaves a lot to be desired in that it has some very significant gaps in mental health care. The one that is most obvious to me lies in the services for the treatment of the chronic, nonfunctional psychiatric patient—specifically, patients with schizophrenia, affective disorder, organic brain disorder, and personality disorder. The methodology and the system to deal with such patients simply does not exist—even though community mental health services were specifically mandated to provide continuity of treatment for this very group of patients [1].

Let me first talk about Dr. Tischler's paper. His objective was to provide hard data (in an area where data was lacking) to evaluate the role of ethnicity in the delivery of mental health services. He discussed parts of five epidemiological (rather than clinical) studies, which looked at ethnicity and the need for care versus the demand for services. Dr. Tischler did both process review and outcome review of cases. He found that, in general, the demand for service matched the group that needed it. He looked at demand in relation to type of service (whether the patients were using full or partial hospitalization versus community, satellite, or ambulatory care services).

He also looked at how services were being used and found that nonwhites had shorter hospital stays and were readmitted more often. This certainly fits in with our own experience that, as best we can determine, those patients with greater family support systems (usually whites rather than nonwhites) will be hospitalized for longer periods of time and, following discharge, will follow treatment recommendations (e.g., taking medication), to a greater degree than those who do not have family support systems. The point is that if one is not taking medication and has a severe psychiatric illness such as schizophrenia, one is much more likely to be hospitalized more often and to leave the hospital earlier. Lastly, Dr. Tischler looked at quality of care and again found that ethnicity was not a factor.

All in all, the data that Dr. Tischler presented tends to be very reassuring. Services do seem to be meeting the needs of different ethnic groups. However, I tend to agree with Dr. Ellsworth that the stronger predictor of whether or not one will obtain services is the severity of one's illness. This will outweigh one's ethnicity. Dr. Tischler is rightly cautious; he warns us that his data are fragmentary, his samples are small, and the patients he is looking at come from only one treatment service. He has not, however, presented a breakdown of his patient population by diagnosis, which I think is crucial in trying to determine whether the demand for services is being met. He also pointed out that the study was done in an actual treatment setting and therefore is not as controlled as he (or I) would like to see.

To summarize, it is important to set up community mental health services to serve not only the needs of particular ethnic groups, but also those of various diagnostic groups. The needs of the patient with neurosis or personality disorder are quite different from the needs of the patient with chronic schizophrenia or chronic organic brain syndrome. This is the message I want to leave and this is the area that Dr. Tischler and his group need to look into further. With that introduction, let me briefly present our work and its relevance to the topic of evaluation. We (Dr. William Hargreaves, myself, and our co-workers) have performed a controlled study of the relative effectiveness of short hospitalization (defined as 21 to 28 days) as an alternative to long hospitalization (90 to 120 days) for psychiatric patients in need of hospital care for whom both treatments are judged clinically feasible (1—5).

Our sample consisted of 235 consecutively admitted voluntary psychiatric patients who were randomly assigned to either short term or long term hospitalization on the same ward. Both groups received intensive treatment using all appropriate modalities and adequate psychopharmacological dosage schedules. Ratings were made during hospitalization and at one and two years after admission, using the Psychiatric Evaluation Form (PEF) to rate symptoms, the Katz Adjustment Scales to rate social functioning, a Historical Information Form to rate role function and to record life history and treatment information, and the Health-Sickness Rating Scale (HSRS) to rate global outcome (Figure 3—7).

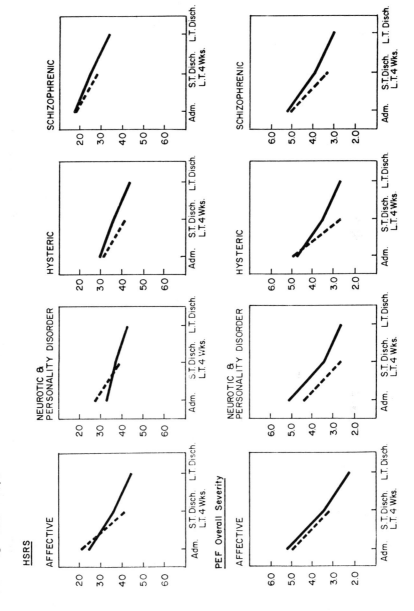

Figure 3–7. Global Outcomes, as Measured by Health-Sickness Rating Scale and PEF Overall Severity Item, for Four Diagnostic Groups

For subjects assigned to the short term group, discharge planning began immediately, with the goal of enabling the patient to leave in three weeks. Strategy for the long term group included a two- to three-week assessment of psychodynamics, precipitants of hospitalization, and clinical diagnosis. Treatment was oriented to long range psychosocial reorganization through psychotherapy, medication, and major rehabilitative measures. A partially fixed drug regimen was used for schizophrenic subjects in an effort to use similarly high phenothiazine levels in both the short term and long term groups during the first 21 days in the hospital.

During the inpatient phase, the short term subjects, both schizophrenic and nonschizophrenic, improved sooner than the long term subjects; that is, short term subjects were functioning significantly better, just prior to their discharge, than were their long term counterparts at four weeks after admission. Schizophrenic and nonschizophrenic long term subjects continued to improve during the remainder of their hospital stay, but only the long term schizophrenic subjects were functioning significantly better when discharged, than were the short term schizophrenic subjects at their earlier time of discharge. Comparison between diagnostic subgroups of nonschizophrenics showed that subjects with affective disorders were mostly severely impaired at admission and subsequently improved most during hospitalization, regardless of length of stay.

We found that at one year following admission, the long term schizophrenic subjects showed significantly better global functioning than did their short term counterparts. This trend persisted, but was not statistically significant at two years following admission. However, long term treatment continued to yield superior global outcome for the subgroup of schizophrenics with relatively good prehospital functioning; that is, there was a statistically significant interaction between treatment assignment and prehospital functioning on all three global outcome measures.

Short term and long term schizophrenic subjects were rehospitalized in about the same number, for approximately the same total number of days during the two-year followup period. There was essentially no difference in global functioning between short and long term nonschizophrenic patients at both one and two years following admission, nor did the two nonschizophrenic groups differ in amount of outpatient treatment received.

The long term schizophrenic subjects received significantly more outpatient psychotherapy than did the short term schizophrenic subjects during the first year post-admission, but not during the second year. The mean monthly amounts of psychotropic medications taken during the posthospital period were greater for long term schizophrenic subjects than for short term schizophrenic subjects. Long term schizophrenic subjects who functioned poorly in the two years before admission received greater mean monthly amounts of posthospital psychotropic medications, than did the long term schizophrenic subjects with better prehospital functioning. For short term schizophrenic subjects there were no obvious differences between subjects with good and poor pre-hospital functioning in the mean monthly amount of psychotropic medication taken during the followup period. At two years post-admission, there were no consistent differences among the groups on symptoms, work, socialization, and family relationships. This was true for both the schizophrenic and nonschizophrenic groups.

The implications of these findings for other treatment settings involve a judgment concerning the cost effectiveness of the two types of treatment. During the inpatient phase, short term subjects generally had an earlier remission of acute symptoms than did the long term subjects. At one year, long term treatment resulted in better global functioning for schizophrenic subjects, while this effect persisted to the second year only within a subgroup of schizophrenics with relatively good pre-hospital functioning. Our hypothesis is that long term treatment may be the treatment of choice for schizophrenic patients with good pre-hospital functioning. Further studies are needed to assess this interaction between treatment and prehospital functioning.

To Summarize

I have discussed Dr. Tischler's paper, I have presented our outcome findings, and I agree, that many of the patients we now treat in community mental health centers are not receiving the services they need. I also agree with Dr. West, that in many ways our money could have been better spent in educating our staffs in the natural history and treatment of the very patients that the community mental health centers serve. Treatment should be based on empirical data rather than on political rhetoric. My suggestion is for a new mental health worker who can deal with the complex needs of the chronic psychiatric patient and the special needs which his ethnic background demands.

Chapter 4

Community Treatment
of Schizophrenia

A Re-evaluation of Theoretical
Assumptions

Gerald L. Klerman

My goal is a re-evaluation of theoretical assumptions of
community psychiatry. In pursuit of this end, I will survey
the research findings as to the community treatment of
schizophrenia to determine which alternative theoretical approaches
best accommodate the findings.

From its inception, community psychiatry has been the arena
for many controversies as to theory and practice. Regarding the
community treatment of schizophrenia, two major sets of theoretical
assumptions or models have been debated; these models may be
broadly labelled as the "medical model" and the "social learning
model." The medical model builds upon the traditions of psychiatry
as part of medicine, and views community psychiatry as the extension of mental health services to patients "ill" with diagnosable
"diseases," but who might not have access to these services because
of barriers of lack of facilities, race, poverty, or geography. The
social learning model challenged the assumptions that mental health
was an extension of medicine and that the recipient of services were
either individuals or "ill."

The proponents of these theoretical models have argued their
positions for over two decades. Now, sufficient clinical and research
experience with community treatment of schizophrenia has accumulated to allow careful delineation of the issues and critical comparison of the relative value of the alternative models.

The limitation of my review to schizophrenia itself embodies one
major assumption of the medical model: that diagnostic groupings

have validity and utility. The practice of diagnosis has been the subject of much controversy; some groups within the community health movement have held strong antidiagnostic and antilabelling attitudes. Among the most extreme of such attitudes are those expressed by Szasz, who claims that schizophrenia is a "myth"; by R.D. Laing, who claims that schizophrenics are victims of an oppressive psychotogenic society; and by Rosenhahn, who claims that in practice, the diagnosis of schizophrenia is fraught with error and adverse social-psychological and moral consequences (Szasz, 1961; Laing, 1967; Rosenhahn, 1973).

The social learning model also includes antidrug and antibiological attitudes. Often the staffs of community mental health centers are involved in ideological debates around the value and safety of drug treatment. This debate has been linked to issues of power. As mentioned by Dr. Mosher, MDs, who are the sole legal dispensers of medication, are often in powerful positions of administrative authority. Many antimental health groups, such as the Scientology church, and many civil libertarians are concerned over the potential abuse of medication, particularly in involuntary hospital settings. Together these issues involving diagnosis, the use of drugs as biological intervention, and medical authority, focus some of the differences between the theoretical assumptions of the medical and social learning approaches.

The community treatment of schizophrenia is one policy area where these issues have gained public attention. Among the many controversial issues generated by the community psychiatry movement in America, the appropriateness, efficacy, and morality of the treatment of schizophrenics in community settings ranks very high. Numerous articles in influential newspapers such as the *New York Times*, *Los Angeles Times*, and the *Boston Globe* attest to the concern of many, that patients formerly treated in large public mental hospitals are being prematurely discharged into communities where inadequate residential and treatment facilities exist.

Other segments of the public are fearful that mental patients may have potential to commit serious crimes, especially involving personal violence. Legislative committees in New York, Massachusetts, Pennsylvania, and California are reviewing mental health policies around deinstitutionalization, another indicator of the considerable controversy as to the wisdom of these policies and the adequacy of resources available for community treatment programs.

Within the mental health professions there are similar differences of opinion and controversies as to the quality of evidence for the efficacy of community treatment and the scientific basis for community mental health programs. The preeminent journal *Science*, in recent years has published articles by Crane and Arnhoff which are critical of the research basis for community mental health policies. Arnhoff in particular has raised the question of the social costs to the family, neighborhood, and community generated by large numbers of disabled and chronic schizophrenic patients discharged into the community. Other clinicians have questioned the gain from patients being placed in urban environments where they are subject to predatory abuse, or being forced into a community where the treatment resources may be inadequate (Arnhoff, 1975; Crane, 1974).

To address these controversies, this paper will review the current research evidence for the efficacy and adverse effects of community treatment of patients and the adequacy of available treatment programs. This paper is based on three sources:

1. A review of the literature, particularly reports of controlled studies on medication, rehabilitation programs, psychosocial treatments, and followup studies.
2. My participation in a number of research projects, including: (a) the NIMH Psychopharmacology Research Branch Service Center "Acute Phenothiazine Study" with Cole and Goldberg (Cole, et al., 1964); (b) the current NIMH—PRB Collaborative Study of Fluphenazine; (c) studies with Reidel on the New Haven project on Utilization Review (Reidel et al., 1971) including a followup study reported by Astrachan, Meyers and Schwartz (Schwartz, et al., 1975); and (d) studies at the Erich Lindemann Mental Health Center on patterns of utilization and followup of schizophrenic patients conducted in concert with J. Barrett (Barrett and Klerman, 1976).
3. My experience as director of two community mental health programs, first at the Connecticut Mental Health Center (1967—1969), and then in Boston at the Erich Lindemann Mental Health Center (1970—1976).

Based on these sources, I regard the community treatment of schizophrenia as a major, unresolved issue of immediate professional and public concern. Schizophrenia is one of the nation's major public health problems, both in terms of the number of patients affected, the chronicity of their disability, and the drain on social and medical resources made by their needs. I am concerned especially with the discrepancy between the available research findings and the enactment of public policy. Available research data are pertinent to public policy, yet a major public policy—deinstitutionalization—was enacted in the absence of adequate research.

This policy area is politically important for the mental health field because it tests our credibility. The community mental health movement was proposed to Congress and many state legislatures about fifteen years ago on the premise that its program would provide an effective and feasible alternative to the state hospital. However, the community psychiatry leadership did not make after care programs mandatory, or require program evaluation. After the program was implemented, many community mental health centers were allowed, even encouraged to expand and diversify their service programs without any requirement that they give priority to the needs of schizophrenics. In many cases, this situation led to programmatic anarchy, and the patient group to have suffered the most has often been the severely ill, for whose benefit this program was initially advocated before Congress. Unless we do a better job in evaluating the public policy implications of community treatment, the credibility of the mental health profession and of the National Institute of Mental Health is at stake.

COMMUNITY TREATMENT OF SCHIZOPHRENIA

In the Public Health Framework

In re-evaluating the alternative theoretical assumptions supporting community psychiatry, I have found it useful to apply some public health concepts which are a subvariant of the medical model (Seigler and Osmond, 1974; Klerman, 1975). Dr. Gruenberg (1966) has proposed that the community treatment of schizophrenia has two distinct aspects: the management of the acute schizophrenic episode; and the problems arising from the discharge into the community of chronic patients who have been institutionalized for long periods. These two issues may be regarded respectively as modes of secondary and tertiary prevention from the public health point of view.

The public health framework makes distinctions among primary, secondary, and tertiary prevention. Primary prevention represents the long term hope that when we know enough about the etiology and pathophysiology of a disorder, we can intervene early. In the case of schizophrenia, I do not think we are anywhere near having such knowledge, and, consequently, talking about primary prevention of schizophrenia is a mere exercise in speculation: the generating of hypotheses rather than their testing or application. Secondary prevention refers to early case finding and active intervention with the goal of reduction of mortality, the reduction of morbidity, and the prevention of residual disability. We do know a good deal about how to intervene in the acute schizophrenic psychotic episode. Tertiary prevention refers to rehabilitation aimed at the reduction of residual disability in individuals already suffering from the disorder. Given these concepts, the community treatment of acute schizophrenia and the policy of deinstitutionalization may be viewed as specific forms of secondary and tertiary prevention.

As a Form of Secondary Prevention

In the 1950s two developments occurred almost simultaneously which revolutionalized the treatment of schizophrenia. The first was the introduction of rauwolfia and the phenothiazines, the first of the so-called tranquilizers. These drugs have provided effective treatments for the symptomatic manifestations of many acute schizophrenic psychoses. They have also contributed to shortened durations of hospitalization and increased percentages of patients discharged from acute episodes.

The second development was the introduction of new psychosocial approaches to the hospital milieu and revised attitudes towards the treatment of schizophrenics. A number of novel policies were introduced, first in Britain and then in the United States, including the "open door" policy, avoidance of seclusion and restraint, implementation of large group techniques such as the therapeutic community, upgrading of the status and training of nonprofessionals, conscious effort at early discharge, efforts to break down administrative and other barriers between the hospital and its community, and involvement of the family—a series of developments that became known as "social psychiatry."

It is unfortunate that these two developments occurred at the same time, since the relative contribution of the two to the reduction of patients resident in mental hospitals and to the improved outlook for the management of acute schizophrenic have been obscured. Since 1955, excellent research efforts have supported the value of drugs and of the new psychosocial methods for treatment of acute schizophrenic illnesses. These studies included:

1. A policy of early discharge: The results of the VA study (Caffey, 1967) and of the studies carried out at the Massachusetts Mental Health Center under the leadership of Greenblatt et al., 1965, Drugs and Social Therapies Project) were important in support of this policy in the U.S.A.

2. The recent studies at the New York State Psychiatric Institute by Herz and Endicott (Herz, Endicott, and Spitzer, 1975) at Langley Porter Neuropsychiatric Institute, and at the University of California at San Francisco (Glick et al., 1976) have demonstrated the value of brief, intensive hospitalization for acute schizophrenics.

3. Day treatment has been demonstrated as an effective alternative to inpatient care (Herz, Endicott, and Spitzer, 1971). The most notable treatment study was the Zwerling study, which indicated that as many as 80 percent of patients usually destined for inpatient treatment could be managed in a day treatment program (Zwerling et al., 1962).

4. Home treatment by nurses was evaluated as an alternative to hospitalization by Pasamanick (1967) and associates in Louisville, described in their award-winning book, *Schizophrenics in the Community*. Intensive home treatment by visiting nurses combined with medication could prevent hospitalization and improve family functioning and symptomatic reduction.

These clinical research studies used quasi-experimental designs and attempted to control new treatment, whether drugs, psychosocial innovations, or their combination, by random assignment or matching of patients.

In addition to these clinical studies, the excellent biometric reports by Kramer and his associates (1969) have documented major shifts in the patterns of utilization and treatment, especially for schizophrenics. Overall, the census in public mental hospitals is down, even though the admissions rate remains high, and the death rate has declined. The duration of hospitalization has decreased, and the percentage of newly admitted schizophrenics, whether first episode or other, who are discharged within one year is over 90 percent, compared to less than 50 percent before 1950.

Changes in the Mental Health Care System

These changes in hospital statistics need to be viewed as part of the larger changes in the U.S. mental health care system. There have been major shifts in the structure of the mental health care system, both quantitatively and qualitatively (Kramer, 1976). Since 1950, episodes of inpatient care per 100,000 of the population the rate of inpatient care episodes under all auspices, has remained fairly constant. While the use of hospitalization for all health services has gone up, the mental health field has kept inpatient care fairly stable. This data are in terms of episodes, not patient days. The duration of episodes has decreased and inpatient utilization has remained essentially constant.

Another significant trend is that within the inpatient utilization sector, there has been a very dramatic change in where patients go when they are hospitalized. The previous governmental monopoly on delivery of psychiatric care has been broken. We now have a pluralistic care system, from which schizophrenics have clearly benefited along with other groups. In 1955, 80 percent of all inpatient care was provided in public mental hospitals, VA, state, or county. In 1973, these public mental hospitals accounted for less than 50 percent of inpatient care episodes. Now, the largest proportion of episodes are treated in community mental health centers or psychiatric units in general hospitals.

A third trend is that while inpatient utilization per 100,000 of population has remained constant, the utilization of outpatient services has skyrocketed. Although psychiatry may be criticized by the antipsychiatrists, the public acts as if it believes in psychiatry as a part of medicine. The public is making use of psychiatric facilities at a rapidly increasing rate per 100,000. These data are only from units reporting to NIMH, which include mental health clinics and child guidance clinics in the public sector. These data do not include care given in the private practice sector, and consequently are an under-representation of the extent to which mental health services are being utilized. In 1973, over 2 percent of the population made use of some mental health facility during the year. If one could obtain data on the use of the private sector, the rates would probably be double that figure.

These trends are paralleled by the rise in outpatient utilization by schizophrenics. Whereas in 1955 almost all care for schizophrenics was on inpatient basis, in 1974 schizophrenics are being treated in the outpatient as well as the inpatient sector. Another way of looking at the same data is to note the significant growth of the outpatient sector from 25 percent of all episodes of care in 1955, to over half of all episodes of care in 1973. Moreover, a completely new form of delivery; the community mental health center, has been created. This new delivery component did not exist before 1965. After less than ten years, the community mental health center accounts for 25 percent of all health care episodes and for about 20 percent of episodes for schizophrenics.

Unanswered Questions Meriting Further Research

Impressive as the gains have been, there remain those unanswered questions.

Does there exist a group of acute schizophrenics for whom medication is not necessary, or perhaps even contraindicated? Mosher (1974) at the NIMH Center for Schizophrenia, and M. Goldstein (1970) at UCLA have suggested that there may well be a significant subgroup of acute schizophrenics, perhaps in the neighborhood of 5 to 15 percent, who do not require phenothiazine treatment, and who may actually be harmed by this treatment. Placebo-controlled studies indicate that while the majority of patients do poorly on placebo, there are a significant group of about 25 to 30 percent who seem to do reasonably well. While the predictors of these good responders are yet unclear, they may correspond to the previous description by Langfeldt (1939) of schizophreniform patients, or in the process-reactive/good premorbid group described by Garmezy (1974) and Rodnick (1973).

Given the likelihood that patients currently diagnosed as schizophrenic represent a heterogeneous group etiologically and clinically, the existence of these patients and other subgroups differentially responsive to pharmacologic and psychologic treatments is highly probable. In our enthusiasm for the intensive treatment of acute episodes, we should not overlook the possibility that significant subgroups exist who might benefit by alternative strategies.

What is the optimal duration of hospital treatment of acute schizophrenic psychoses? In almost all studies of hospitalization, the assumption has been that "less is better," and that there is an inverse linear relationship between duration of hospitalization and outcome. This view is based on extrapolation from very good studies, particularly the VA studies and the sociological studies of Goffman (1961) in the United States and Brown et al. (1966) in Great Britain, documentating the deleterious effects of long term hospitalization. However, some recent evidence suggests that very brief hospital treatment (less than 30 days) may not be optimal. It is not clear if this is due to the duration of the hospital treatment period itself, or to the adequacy of aftercare. Weissman et al. (1969), working at the Connecticut Mental Health Center while I was Director, reported their experiences in a unit where there was an administrative limitation of five days' duration of stay. A followup of patients treated on that ward indicated that the nonschizophrenics did well with the five-day maximum. However, a high proportion of the schizophrenics were rehospitalized within a few months.

The optimum hospitalization for the acute episode is not established. We need to regard the duration of hospitalization as akin to the dosage of a drug. It may well be that prolonged hospitalization has adverse effects; but there probably is a threshold period below which too brief a hospitalization provides inadequate duration of time for medication regulation, initiation of rehabilitation programs, reconstitution of a psychotic episode, renegotiation of family relations, and so forth.

What proportion of patients become chronic after an acute episode? The vast majority of acute patients do improve and are discharged. However, up to 15 percent of patients become chronically hospitalized within one to two years. This phenomenon was called "silting" by Kraft and his associates at Ft. Logan (1971). In our experience at the Erich Lindemann Mental Health Center in Boston, the rate was about 5 percent (Klerman and Barrett, unpublished data, 1976).

The NIMH—PSC Collaborative Study indicated about 5 percent of a selected group of drug-treated patients did not improve. The most impressive evidence of this phenomenon comes from the studies of Smith and associates in Illinois, (1974), who compared a cohort of acute schizophrenics treated at a mental health center with those treated at the nearby state hospital. The results for the immediate outcome indicated some superiority for the intensive treatment at the community mental health center, but at the end of one year there were residual groups of disabled patients of equal magnitude (about 10—15 percent) at both institutions. These patients represent the failure of current treatment of acute episodes; they require intensive or more long term rehabilitative efforts.

Why is there a lag in the incorporation of demonstrated efficacious innovations into the treatment program? Some techniques, such as new drugs, are readily accepted. The number of day hospitals remains amazingly small, and the number of home treatment programs is infinitesimal; yet the controlled studies in their support are good. The vast majority of acute psychotic episodes are still treated in hospitals, even if they are mental health centers or psychiatric units in general hospitals. Although the research evidence is very good (from the Pasamanick studies and the Zwerling studies) that both home treatment and day programs can be highly effective, neither has been incorporated into many regular treatment programs.

Do health insurance regulations reinforce hospitalization and deter the use of alternatives? Is there resistance within the profession? Does the profession not really accept certain research findings? What would be the optimum mix in an ideal program including hospitalization, home treatment, day programs, emergency room treatment, etc.? To determine the answers to the above questions requires not only controlled trials, but also program evaluation of a more complex nature than most current research efforts can easily mount.

Deinstitutionalization As Tertiary Prevention

It is of interest that while research efforts have documented the value of short term hospitalization and alternatives to hospitalization for acute episodes, the most far-reaching policy implications were felt by the chronically hospitalized patients in large mental hospitals. In the last decade, almost every state's department of mental health instituted the policy of discharging previously chronically hospitalized patients. A number of conferences have recently been held on the closing of state hospitals (Greenblatt, 1974), and some observers have predicted the forthcoming end of the state hospital system. California has probably gone the furthest with this policy. Massachusetts, for example, has already seen the closing of three state hospitals out of a total of twelve, and plans are underway for the possible closing of two more. Nationwide, there has been a major reduction in the number of patients resident in mental hospitals.

To a great extent, these figures are deceptive. A major proportion of the reduction of the census of patients resident in public mental hospitals is a result of the movement of elderly mentally ill patients from mental hospitals into nursing homes, as pointed out by Kramer and his associates (1976). This shift results in an improvement in the statistics of the mental health agencies, and has probably contributed to an improvement in the status of the budgets of state departments of mental health, since the fiscal burden of care for patients in nursing homes is borne by Medicare and other federally supported programs.

Whether transfer of patients to nursing homes contributes to the quality of their life and their longevity is not clear. There are data that the opposite is true; that mentally ill patients transferred to nursing homes have fared poorly, with less opportunities for socialization and recreation, less sophisticated use of medication, and an increase in mortality due to the psychosocial and psychobiological trauma of transfer itself—as well as to the uneven, if not actually poor, quality of medical care in many nursing homes.

In addition to the decline in census due to shifts of patients to nursing homes, a large proportion of the decline in census is accounted for by the discharge of many patients into the community. It is this policy, called "deinstitutionalization," which has generated the most controversy. Research evidence in direct support of this policy is difficult to find. Whereas excellent studies have documented the value of brief hospitalization and community alternatives to hospitalization for the treatment of acute psychoses, I cannot find comparable studies of similar quality comparing groups of patients placed in the community with matched groups remaining in state or VA hospitals. Deinstitutionalization became a slogan and de facto policy, in my opinion, based on limited research evidence.

Deinstitutionalization as Public Policy

The policy of deinstitutionalization fostered an interesting alliance of three groups. One group included progressive leaders in the mental health field who extrapolated from research demonstrating the value of outpatient treatment for acute episodes, and reasoned that what was good for acute schizophrenics would be good for chronic schizophrenics. The second group included civil libertarians, who were genuinely concerned with the abuses of "total institution." The third group included the fiscal conservatives in states such as California, who felt that there was budgetary gain in transferring hospitalized patients into community settings where they would be under the aegis of public welfare agencies, rather than the responsibility of the departments of mental health. This policy had very little research evidence in its support. I cannot find any systematic study evaluating a group of chronically hospitalized patients placed in community facilities compared to a matched group treated in a good, well equipped rehabilitation hospital unit.

This major public policy decision was almost simultaneously made in about 40 states between 1965 and 1970, with a consequential discharge of very large numbers of patients into urban and rural communities. The policy, like many, was made in the absence of data. Two types of data are needed. First, we need data as to the limits of community care—i.e., under the optimum circumstances, how far could we go in community care, not for acute patients, but for chronic patients, those hospitalized for two continuous years? Second, what actually occurs in under less than optimum conditions? Most care and treatment in institutions and communities is less than optimal.

What is unclear is the relative cost benefit of the policy of deinstitutionalization. We have relatively few followup studies of patients in the community. Some studies have been done in California; their findings are disheartening. There are now two unpublished followup studies of patients from Grafton State Hospital, which closed in Massachusetts (Khan, 1975). Most studies indicate that, at a minimum, 50 percent of chronic patients living in the community are markedly socially isolated and in marginal rates. They require fiscal

subsidy via disability assistance and/or welfare. They reside in boarding homes, nursing homes or under other forms of foster care where
for the most part they have minimum opportunities for socialization.

The observations of Murphy (1976) in Canada and newspaper articles in New York raise the serious question as to the adequacy of
provisions for their safety and for the protection of their financial
resources and personal security. The adequacy of followup care is
often minimal, and the "revolving door" phenomenon is well known.

Research on Combining Drugs
and Psychosocial Therapies

In reviewing the literature on optimum care, the best research
efforts have been on combinations of drugs and psychosocial treatment. There are good studies of the value of medication in after care.
Davis (1975) reviewed 23 controlled studies evaluating the value of
maintenance antipsychotic treatment in chronic patients either in an
institution or in the community. He concludes that evidence was
overwhelmingly positive for value of drug therapy. Davis did not
review the evidence for combined treatment.

The best study of combined treatment was conducted in Baltimore by Hogarty and Goldberg (1973). Patients were treated with
drugs alone versus placebo alone, plus some form of social therapy
and compared. The evidence was very good that drugs alone were
better than placebo, and also that psychosocial treatment was a significant contribution to drug therapy. For patients on phenothiazine
medication, the rehospitalization rate is significantly reduced. The
greatest reduction occurred for those patients who were diligent in
taking their medication, and for those whose medication was combined with psychosocial therapy aimed at facilitating their ongoing
social adjustment.

The advent of long-acting depot fluphenazine has greatly contributed to patient compliance. The work of Leff and Wing and their
associates (1971) in London indicates the profound and complex
interactions of drug treatment, the type of family and residential
setting in which the patient lives, and the support of mental health
services in increasing the schizophrenic patient's capacity to cope
with stress and sustain him/herself in the community.

With schizophrenics, psychotherapy is secondary or contingent
upon the prior symptom reduction derived from drug therapy. I call
this the "two-stage rocket theory" of combined treatment. In the
first stage, drug treatment is a necessary but not always sufficient
component of a comprehensive treatment program. Drugs get patients out of the gravitational field of symptoms, and having done so,

the patients can then benefit from psychotherapeutic methods such as group therapy, social work, or vocational rehabilitation. Psychotherapy effects are second in time as well as in the sense that efficacy is contingent upon prior symptom reduction. Also, psychotherapy acts on different outcome variables than do drugs: drugs reduce symptoms while psychotherapy improves personal adjustment. This view of combined therapy is most applicable to after care of schizophrenics in the community.

The accessibility of schizophrenics to social intervention is not linear, but rather an inverted *U* related to the degree of symptomatic distress. Venables (1967) has related response to level of autonomic arousal. Patients who are very high in symptomatic distress in the psychotic range are less accessible to psychosocial interventions. The function of drugs is to move patients into the right side of the curve. In this concept, patients who are very high in arousal and have high degrees of overt symptomatology are inaccessible to the usual forms of psychosocial learning, especially psychotherapy. Medication moves patients into the low arousal range. The concern here, however, is if patients are moved into too low arousal, they become "psychosocial zombies," a condition that has been described in newspaper reports of the overmedicated patients found in many after care programs.

The Actual Conditions of Treatment

Unfortunately, when we review data on actual practice in community treatment for schizophrenics, the findings are bleak. As Hogarty (1971) has documented, the gap between the existing research findings and actual practice is immense. Surveys recently undertaken to determine the quality of life of schizophrenics residing in public mental hospitals indicate that there are appalling degrees of dehumanization and deindividualization.

Whatever the criticisms applicable to Rosenhan's conclusions pertaining to diagnosis and the medical model (Spitzer, 1975), we cannot ignore the findings of his and other studies documenting the impersonality of mental hospitals and the tendency of staff members to disregard the individual needs of patients. Although the census of state mental hospitals has decreased greatly, the quality of treatment has not significantly improved. The available data indicate that patients residing in public mental hospitals still receive poor treatment. The phenomenon of institutionalization identified by Goffman and other sociologists in the 1950s continues to prevail.

The situation, unfortunately, is little better for patients in the community. New forms of community chronicity have been developed in many large urban settings such as New York, Chicago, Los

Angeles, and San Francisco. In the absence of an adequate network of after care facilities, community residences, halfway houses, sheltered workshops, and day treatment centers, large numbers of patients are relegated to "lives of quiet desperation" in welfare hotels, and in segregated neighborhoods. They are subsisting on minimal incomes from social welfare or disability payments, and receiving poorly monitored, often poorly prescribed psychotropic medication.

Comparison of this picture with the potential demonstrated by imaginative research programs in the 1950s and 1960s, is appalling. Research studies such as those by Gruenberg (1962), Fairweather (1969), by the Fountain House group in New York, and others indicate that the combination of antipsychotic drug medication plus the availability of a network of property supervised rehabilitative, vocational and residential facilities could reduce the disability and social isolation of schizophrenics.

The promise of the community mental health program has been only partially realized. Application of the available knowledge failed to materialize except in a few selected community mental health centers. Perhaps the mental health movement was overambitious and expanded its responsibility too quickly, into the realms of alcoholism, drug abuse, racism, and social unrest, without being sure that the problems of the schizophrenics—one of our primary clinical obligations—had been met. Perhaps it has been a failure of the National Institute of Mental Health to assign priority and resources to this need. Perhaps it has been an overestimation of the extent to which community attitudes had in fact changed. Whatever the reasons, the community treatment of schizophrenic remains an area of high relevance but low success (Klerman, 1974).

THE LIMITS OF COMMUNITY PSYCHIATRY

Attempts at reform of mental institutions, even when successful (as with the therapeutic community movement within the mental hospital), have only partially satisfied the critics and skeptics. In their demands for redress of social grievances, professionals such as Szasz and Laing, jurists such as Bazalon, and lawyers representing the public interest such as Helperin, have joined with spokesmen for the new left, black militants, and even some right wing conservatives in criticizing mental hospitals as being both ineffective and unjust. Their remedy is radical—deinstitutionalization, the dismantling of these institutions. Decarceration is the battle cry of the new abolitionists.

These critics argue that the ineffectiveness of the mental institutions results only in part from the unintended consequences of their internal organization which undermine the otherwise noble attempts of staff at rehabilitation and treatment. According to these critics, attempts at therapeutic change within the mental institution are only partial solutions. The feature of total institutions leading most inescapably to their failure, they assert, is not so much the internal organization of the total institutions as their relationship to the larger society, that is, their role as "double agents."

Modern mental institutions claim commitment to both social control and to personal change; yet whenever conflicts arise between the two goals, the social control mandate usually takes priority. Why? Because it is claimed that ultimately the public mental hospital is under the legal aegis, administrative control, and fiscal support of the society and its legislatures, commissions, and agencies whose highest priority is controlling deviance rather than meeting the needs of the individual patients.

The community mental health movement gained public recognition in the 1960s with President Kennedy's message to Congress. The creation of day care centers, halfway houses, community residences, and rehabilitation programs began in the mental health field. These reforms have had marked success. In contrast to the prisons, whose populations are growing and where internal discontent is great, the mental hospitals have seen a reduction in resident population and a radical restructuring of their place in the mental health care delivery system. The structure of the mental health care delivery system has changed. The majority of mentally ill patients are now being treated as outpatients. In 1950, 80 percent of all mental health episodes were treated in public hospitals; today, the public hospital provides the minority of treatment episodes. For inpatient treatment, psychiatric units in general hospitals and private hospitals, rather than public mental health institutions, are providing the settings for the majority of admissions.

The mental health system has experienced a major shift away from almost total reliance upon public institutions employing involuntary incarceration and treatment, towards a voluntaristic and pluralistic system. The shift has been to a voluntaristic system because increasing numbers of patients have the choice of going for treatment; the system has become pluralistic as patients gain more options for the type of treatment that they will receive. No longer is the mental health system a state government owned and operated monopoly, as is still the case with correctional institutions. The availability of increased numbers of individual practitioners, nonprofit hospitals, and voluntary agencies has greatly diversified the treatment alternatives. The availability of a voucher system, in the form of health insurance, gives the patient and his or her family, increasing degrees of freedom.

But, the mental health field is experiencing a backlash in both legislatures and local communities. In the case of community mental health, many neighborhoods are resisting placement of halfway houses, community residences, and day programs in their area. While resistance to the placement of patients in the community has been anticipated, an unexpected consequence of deinstitutionalization has been the emergence of new forms of chronicity. Community chronicity is emerging as a major unforeseen problem for the mentally ill (Klerman, 1976).

These reflections upon backlash and chronicity as problems for community mental health are intended to place current controversies in some perspective. We do not know how to gauge the capacity or willingness of the society, or even of individual neighborhoods, to tolerate, accept, and integrate deviant behavior. In practice, the limits of community acceptance are determined by trial and error, with periods of reform followed by retrenchment, usually with a return to some form of institutionalization.

One outgrowth of an appraisal of mental hospitals and other total institutions is the insight that the opportunity for greatest individual freedom is found in a social system where we can choose which of our multiple roles are played with which persons and in what locales. Thus the large modern city, with its opportunities of multiple personal groupings and freedom of movement, is potentially far more individualistic than the small rural village or the commune. However, in the city, we also find counter forces which limit our individuality; ironically, the price often paid for the city's potential for freedom of choice is actual social isolation.

In fact, personal loneliness characterizes much of modern urban life, especially for the poor, the marginal, and the mentally ill. Thus the urban community may generate exactly the same psychological consequences that Goffman identified in the total institution; it is very possible that one of the unintended consequences of decarceration and deinstitutionalization may be new forms of anomie and isolation for the schizophrenic in the community (Klerman, 1975).

CONCLUSIONS

The community psychiatry movement has been the arena for multiple theoretical conflicts. Among the most active controversies have been those around the medical model; various other models have also been proposed, including the social learning model. In this paper I have examined the evidence regarding the community treatment of schizophrenics, and concluded that the most appropriate way to view the current data is from the public health variant of the medical model. In the public health approach, efforts at intervention are divided into primary, secondary, and tertiary preventions. Since we know relatively little about etiology, our efforts at primary prevention are purely speculative.

Current efforts in the community treatment of schizophrenia can be divided into those which aim at secondary prevention and those which aim at tertiary prevention. In the area of secondary prevention is the intensive treatment of the acute psychotic episode, aimed at early case finding, rapid, intensive intervention with drugs, psychosocial methods, and other techniques, which aim at reduction of mortality and morbidity, and the prevention of disability. In tertiary prevention efforts, the aim is to reduce disability in patients already afflicted and to promote their rehabilitation. In these efforts we are failing considerably, and the controversy around deinstitutionalization underscores the lack of adequate knowledge, both as to the limits of available techniques and as to the extent to which current knowledge is being applied.

This public health model can be contrasted to the social learning model which was offered in the early days of the community mental health movement as an alternative to the medical model. Many advocates of the social learning model expressed antidiagnosis attitudes, in which case the separation of schizophrenics would be regarded as theoretically invalid and morally inappropriate. Others were antibiological, and resisted the therapeutic use of drugs. The evidence from the community treatment of schizophrenia supports the validity of the public health model against the social learning model. The social learning model would not deal adequately with the special needs of the schizophrenic, and would deprive the schizophrenic of the benefits of the sick role. The antibiological attitudes of the social learning model would have further deprived the schizophrenics of the benefits of drug treatment, even acknowledging their limitations.

The research evidence indicates that while intensive treatment of acute episodes is a very good means for secondary prevention, the scientific basis for deinstitutionalization as a public policy for tertiary prevention remains inadequate. Deinstitutionalization was implemented in many states as public policy in the 1960s. This policy was based on minimal research evidence, on extrapolation from the studies on acute patients, and also from the deleterious effects of chronic hospitalization. These extrapolations were not automatically true; in other words, just because community treatment prevents chronicity does not mean that it automatically reverses the chronic disabilities of long institutionalized patients.

Nor do the obvious deleterious effects of chronic hospitalization automatically lead to the romantic view that any kind of community treatment will eradicate the illness of schizophrenia. The sociologic studies of the deleterious effects of institutionalism, and other consequences of mental hospitals, led many to believe that all the chronic schizophrenia was the consequence of an adverse institutional social structure.

Now we are in the position that research is necessary after the fact of policy formulation. More work is needed on the interactions between drugs and psychosocial methods of treatment to document the additive and interactive models. More important is the need for research on the quality of care for patients in the community so as to better guide the development of public policy.

What is most needed, however, is national leadership at scientific and professional levels. The credibility of the mental health movement is in danger of being undermined. The community mental health program was instituted in large part because of promises made that it would be directed to the special needs of chronically hospitalized patients. Failure to assign high priority to the needs of these patients can only be interpreted by the public as a failure of both our moral and professional leadership.

Functioning and Stress of Schizophrenics in Community Adjustment

George Serban

The shift of focus of therapeutic intervention from institutional care to community-based services, heralded as a major revolution in the approach to the treatment of schizophrenics, apparently fell short of its expectations. Despite various modalities of immediate therapeutic intervention at the community level, such as crisis intervention, partial hospitalization, halfway houses, and vocational rehabilitation, the high rate of rehospitalizations for schizophrenics seems to be minimally affected, remaining at a fairly constant level of 34 percent.

With the emphasis directed to various forms of community intervention in order to forestall the rehospitalization of chronic schizophrenics, little attention has been paid in research to the real level of schizophrenics' functioning and adjustment in the community. The assessment of community integration is based primarily on evidence of some level of social activities these patients have shown in a community setting, and defined, thereby, as their community adjustment. In general, the criteria of adjustment were reduced to employment vs. unemployment, marital adjustment vs. single, or degree of participation in various community programs, when in reality these data hardly reflect the true adjustment for the majority of schizophrenics who are on welfare, unmarried, or peripherally involved in the social life of the community.

This limited instrumental functioning, derived from the classical criteria of social competence (Turner and Zabo, 1968; Zigler and Phillips, 1967), gives only a fragmented indication for the measurement of adaptation of schizophrenics in the community since it fails to show all the facets of the schizophrenics' psychosocial functioning and, as such, the real level of functioning (if any) in the community setting. In addition, this approach does not specify the particular factors in patients' functioning responsible for the difficulty in adjusting to the community. Furthermore, they omit the evaluation of stress experienced by the patient at that particular level of adaptation.

If in clinical terms community adjustment reflects patients' social and interpersonal functioning when extrapolated for research, the adjustment represents a product of interaction between his level of functioning and the amount of stress he is able to absorb. In the past these two factors had been reduced to social competence, derived itself from premorbid social functioning and stressful precipitating events; only recently had attempts been made to assess their full impact in the community adjustment of schizophrenics. One such attempt was made by Micheaux et al. (1969) in a one-year followup study, but the stress variable was not measured except for precipitating events.

Yet the assumption that inability to maintain tenure in the community is related only to acute precipitating events, which allegedly lead to rehospitalization (Birley and Brown, 1970), does not necessarily have any specific relevance to the actual reason for the schizophrenics' impaired functioning in the community (Serban, 1975b). Actually, the need for rehospitalization was always the result of the schizophrenics' inability to cope with societal demands in an area either of social performance, and/or family interaction and interpersonal relationships, which implicitly assumes generalized stress, not necessarily related specifically to a particular area of disturbed behavior and functioning.

Nevertheless, clinical stress as such has not been adequately measured until recently. Although various theories of the etiology of schizophrenia have acknowledged its role as a main factor for some time (Epstein and Cole), various scales related to stress measured essentially the intensity of stress as major events affecting individual life (Dohrenwend, 1974; Holmes and Rahe, 1967; Langner and Michel, 1963; Micheaux, Katz et al., 1968; Philips, 1953; Wallis, 1972). In general, these scales either tend to measure stress in too general terms or permit the interviewer too much subjectivity in the interpretation of the patient's responses. It is also important to note that all these scales reflect a failure to recognize the possibility that functioning and stress are interacting, influencing each other positively or negatively and thus should be measured simultaneously.

Attempts at measurement in the past have generally treated functioning and stress as unrelated phenomena. In this respect social adjustment sclaes—i.e., the Elgin Prognostic Scale (1944), the Phillips Prognostic Rating Scale (1953), and the Ullman-Giovannoni Scale (1964) basically attempt to predict long term outcome as related to premorbid functioning (except for the Katz Assessment Scale, which predicts rehospitalization only on a basis of several life situation variables). The disadvantage of most of these scales lies in their potentially distorted reliability produced by complete dependency on case history data, the possible bias introduced by raters, and their reported incongruency with patient self-ratings (Magaro, 1968; Watson and Logue, 1968).

In general, these scales attempt to tap primarily factors related to the reactive-process distinction rather than the level of patients' functioning within one year prior to his hospitalization. It should be emphasized at this point that no systematic attempts have been made with these scales to compare the schizophrenic functioning under stress with that of comparable normals for a determined period prior to hospitalization.

The aim of the present investigation was to answer three principal questions resulting from the complete study of the levels of functioning and stress in schizophrenics. The first question referred to the level of functioning of schizophrenics compared to that of normals from the same catchment area and the same sociodemographic background. The second question dealt with the amount of stress that schizophrenics experienced in their adjustment to life in the community before hospitalization, as compared with normals. Pertaining to it is the issue of the interaction between levels of stress and functioning in both the schizophrenic and the normal population within their community adjustment, which has to be answered. The third question is an attempt to evaluate the possible contribution of various areas of poor psychosocial functioning as major or contributing stressors to the rehospitalization of schizophrenics.

METHOD

Sample

A sample of 904 schizophrenic patients was randomly selected from the schizophrenic population at Bellevue, from which alcoholics, drug addicts, and mentally retarded subjects with schizophrenic reaction were screened. The patients were diagnosed at admission as schizophrenics and the diagnoses were re-evaluated by the ward psychiatrists. They were reexamined independently on admission to the project by a staff psychiatrist with the Problem Appraisal Scale (PAS, Spitzer and Endicott, 1969) and diagnosed in accordance with DSM II (APA, 1968).

The agreement rate for diagnosis of subtype schizophrenia was 75 percent for schizo-affective, 83.3 percent for paranoid, 88.2 percent for undifferentiated and 83.3 percent for latent schizophrenia. This distribution of diagnostic groups in these four subclassifications were tested by means of a 2×4 contingency table. The resulting X^2 of 5.10 ($df = 3, p > .05$) shows no differences between the classification of the psychiatrists. For the chronic sample the diagnosis agreement rate was respectively 90.2, 90.7, 92.9, and 75 percent. The X^2 test for the 2×4 diagnostic array was 1.03 ($df = 3$), indicating no difference between the raters.

The sample population was further reduced to 641 schizophrenics through the course of the study because of release from the hospital, refusal to cooperate, and the discovery, later on, of misdiagnosis of schizophrenia as a principal diagnosis. The acutes were defined as only first hospitalization cases without previous treatment of more than three months in any psychiatric setup. In order to eliminate any possible confusion with chronics, it was not based upon any arbitrary number of hospitalizations.

The acute sample consisted of 125 subjects of whom 17 (13.6 percent) were schizo-affective, 43 (34.4%) paranoid, 50 (40%) schizophrenic episode, 2 (1.6%) catatonic, 13 (10.4%) other types. The chronic sample, defined by multiple hospitalizations consisted of 516 subjects of whom 63 (12.2%) were schizo-affective, 192 (37.2%) paranoid, 245 (47.5%) chronic undifferentiated type, 1 (0.2%) catatonic, and 15 (2.9%) other types. Of the acutes, 97 (77.6%) had a sudden onset ranging from one week or less up to three months before first hospitalization, while for 28 (22.4%) the onset ranged from over three months up to one year. For the 516 chronic, amount of hospitalization in state hospitals for the last ten years ranged from one to two years; the average number of previous hospitalizations was 3.63.

The tested population represented approximately 0.45 percent of the U.S. schizophrenics admitted to inpatient facilities in 1970 (Taube and Readick, 1972), and 5 percent of the New York State first admission and readmission to state hospitals. From the point of view of the Hollingshead and Redlich Socioeconomic Classification Index, the sample could be considered as falling mainly in groups IV and V (Hollingshead and Redlich, 1958). A comparable group of 95 normals served as controls. The normal sample was selected from community agencies and working places in the Bellevue catchment area. All controls volunteered for this study, and were free from any evidence of psychotic symptomatology or psychiatric hospitalizations. The distribution of sociodemographic characteristics of the patient and normal samples are presented in Table 4–1.

Examination of Table 4—1 reveals that in terms of age, education, and race the samples are comparable. As regards the sex distribution, there was a predominance of males in the schizophrenic sample as compared with the normal controls. However, when sex was regressed on the stress and functioning variables, no significant differences were found. As may be expected, a larger proportion of schizophrenics than normals were single. Within the age range used, schizophrenic marriage rates are considerably below those of normals. In terms of occupation, acutes and normals appear to be comparable. The discrepancy in the chronic sample appears to be accounted for by the drop in occupational level as a function of the duration of illness, especially in view of the fact that occupation refers to job titles held within six months prior to admission. However, it is important to note that no significant differences were noticed among the samples in terms of age ($X^2 = 0.94$, $p > 0.05$), occupation ($X^2 = 2.05$, $p > 0.05$), race ($X^2 = 3.81$, $p > 0.05$), or education ($X^2 = 5.44$, $p > 0.05$).

From the original sample 349 chronics and 70 acutes were available for followup for a period of two years. Of the 349 chronics, 258 (73.9%) were readmitted, while 91 (26.1%) were nonhospitalized. Of the 70 acutes followed up, 31 (44.3%) were readmitted, while 39 (55.7%) were not. Although 32.4 percent of the chronics and 44 percent of the acutes could not be traced in the followup, the remaining sample of 49 patients, which had been followed up, was found to be representative of the original population in terms of age ($X^2 = 3.4$, $p > 0.05$), sex distribution ($X^2 = 1.10$, $p > 0.05$), education ($X^2 = 1.12$, $p > 0.05$), and marital status ($X^2 = 1.71$, $p > 0.05$). In terms of occupational level, a larger proportion of the followed-up population was represented by unskilled categories.

Technique of Measurement

The measures of social and interpersonal functioning and stress were derived from Social Stress and Functionability Inventory for Psychotic Disorders (SSFIPD). The inventory was standardized on 130 schizophrenics and normals at Bellevue Hospital and was shown to clearly differentiate between these two groups (Serban, 1975).

The Inventory provides information regarding psychiatric history, sociodemographic factors, genetic and personality variables associated with the development of illness, and data pertaining to social functioning and associated stress subsumed under the following four areas: Social performance (6 dimensions called categories: education, job, housekeeping, dependence on welfare, management of finances,

Table 4–1. Sociodemographic Characteristics of the Schizophrenic and Normal Samples

Variable	Chronic		Acute		Total Pts.		Normal		X^2
	N	%	N	%	N	%	N	%	
Age									0.94
25	120	23.3	57	45.6	176	27.5	27	28.4	
25–44	352	68.2	62	49.6	414	64.6	58	61.1	
45+	44	8.5	6	4.8	50	7.8	10	10.5	
Sex									9.01*
Male	329	63.8	65	52.0	394	61.5	43	45.3	
Female	187	36.2	60	48.0	247	38.5	52	54.7	
Total	516		125						
Education (in grades)									5.44
7–11	218	42.2	42	33.6	260	40.6	31	32.6	
12	186	36.1	48	38.4	234	36.5	32	33.7	
13+	112	21.7	35	28.0	147	22.9	32	33.7	
Occupation									2.01
Never employed	15	2.9	8	6.4	23	3.5	3	3.2	
Manual workers	281	54.5	55	44.0	335	52.3	43	45.3	
Unskilled	230	44.6	41	32.8	271	42.3	16	16.8	
Semiskilled	51	9.9	13	10.4	64	10.0	27	28.4	
Skilled workers	28	5.4	6	4.8	34	5.3	5	5.2	
Intermediate level	161	31.2	45	36.0	206	32.1	34	35.8	
Owner, small bus.	2	0.3	1	0.8	3	0.5	1	1.0	
Technician	18	3.5	3	2.4	21	3.3	3	3.2	
Salesman	14	2.7	3	2.4	17	2.7	2	2.1	
Clerks	106	20.5	27	2.16	133	20.8	22	23.2	
Semiprofessional	21	4.1	11	8.8	32	5.0	6	6.3	

	n	%	n	%	n	%	n	%	x^2
Higher level	31	6.0	11	8.8	42	6.6	10	10.5	
Administration	13	2.5	5	4.0	18	2.8	1	1.0	
Lesser professional	16	3.2	4	3.2	20	3.1	9	9.5	
Owner, medium bus.	1	0.2	0	0.0	1	0.2	0	0.0	
Manager	0	0.0	1	0.8	2	0.3	0	0.0	
Marital Status									45.94#
Single	306	59.3	80	64.0	386	60.2	25	26.3	
Married	67	13.0	20	16.0	87	13.6	34	35.8	
Separated	143	27.7	25	20.0	168	26.2	36	37.9	
Race									3.81
White	292	56.6	60	48.0	352	54.9	42	44.2	
Black	192	37.2	57	45.6	249	38.9	33	34.7	
Puerto Rican	22	4.3	5	4.0	27	4.2	17	17.9	
Oriental	1	0.2	2	1.6	3	0.5	1	1.1	
Other	9	1.7	1	0.8	10	1.5	2	2.1	

* $p < .01$
# $p < .001$

living circumstances); Family interaction (4 dimensions: relationship to parents, relatives, marital partner and children); Social interpersonal interaction (7 dimensions: dating, sex, relationship with close friends, neighbors, community at large, use of leisure time and religion); Social maladaptive activities (4 dimensions: drinking, use of addictive and psychedelic drugs, anti-social acts). A total of 21 categories of functioning and 21 categories of stress were independently assessed. (See Appendix A and B for a general description of items comprising the 21 categories—pages 239 and 243.)

Social functioning, represented by 174 items, was measured in terms of the level of the individual's ability to fulfill his needs in relationship to the four general areas outlined above (Serban, 1975). Stress, measured by 130 items, reflected the degree of imbalance between environmental demands for psychosocial performance and the capacity for successful fulfillment of these demands (Serban, 1975).

Answers to each item within each of the 21 functioning categories were rated: (1) if they reflected nonfunctioning, (2) if they reflected low functioning, and (3) if they indicated adequate functioning. Answers to each item within each of the 21 stress categories were rated: (1) if they reflected high stress, (2) if they reflected low stress, and (3) if they reflected no stress. The sum of these raw scores was then divided by the number of items rated and thus a mean score for each category of functioning and of stress was derived. This mean score (henceforth referred to as a D score) was computed to compensate for unequal numbers of items in the 21 functioning and stress categories.

Interrater reliability of the inventory was measured in terms of per cent agreement and was found to range between 85 and 91 percent. The SSFIPD was also given by an independent interviewer to an informant (a member of the family such as parent, sibling, spouse, or an individual who lived with the patient during a six-month period prior to his hospitalization). The percent agreement for factual information computed for 228 patients and their informants ranged from 83—91 percent.

The test-retest reliability, determined by Pearsonian correlation (six months interval) for the functioning scores on 7 dimensions reflecting 40 percent factual data (education, job, living condition, marriage, welfare, drinking) and 60 percent attitudinal data, computed for 78 cases, ranged from 0.43 through 0.77. The seven dimensions were: education, job, welfare, dependence, drinking, use of psychedelic and addictive drugs, and antisocial behavior. The tests were individually administered by either project psychiatrists or PhD clinical psychologists, in the wards of Bellevue Hospital, only to patients in contact with their surroundings. The patients were interviewed 3 to 5 days prior to their discharge. All patients were receiving thorazine regularly during hospitalization.

RESULTS

Functioning

As a first step in the data analysis the means and standard deviations of the D functioning scores in each of the 21 categories of the SFFIPD were computed. This was done separately for the normals and the acutes and chronic schizophrenics. A grand mean (mean of the mean D functioning scores across all 21 categories for all subjects within a group) was also computed for each group. Table 4–2 presents these statistics.

An examination of the group means reveals a general tendency for the normals to show higher levels of functioning than the schizophrenics, and for the acute schizophrenics to show higher levels than the chronic patients. In order to determine the significance of these differences, analyses of variance that compared the three groups on functioning were computed for each of the 21 categories and for the mean of these categories. Results of these analyses are presented in Table 4–3. They show that the three groups were significantly different on 16 of the 21 categories (Education, Job, Welfare, Finance, Living Circumstances, Parents, Relatives, Marriage, Children, Dating, Sex, Friends, Neighbors, Leisure, Addictive Drugs, Antisocial Acts) and the mean of the categories.

In order to determine which of the group differences contributed significantly to the overall differences obtained among the means, the Scheffé method (Scheffé, 1957) for individual mean comparisons was applied. The resulting F tests were computed for differences between normals and acutes, normals and chronics, and chronics and acutes. Table 4–3 presents the results of these comparisons. The normal subjects showed significantly higher levels of functioning than the acutes on 14 categories and on the grand mean of the categories (Education, Job, Living Circumstances, Parents, Marriage, Children, Dating, Sex, Friends, Others, Leisure, Drinking, Addictive Drugs, and Antisocial Acts).

Finally, in contrasting acutes and chronics, it was found that acutes surpassed chronics significantly on 13 categories of functioning and on the grand mean of all the functioning categories (Education, Job, Welfare, Finances, Parents, Relatives, Marriage, Dating, Friends, Neighbors, Others, Leisure, and Antisocial Acts). In general,

Table 4–2.   Means and Standard Deviations of D Function Scores for Normals and Acute and Chronic Schizophrenics on the 21 Functioning Categories

Category	Normals			Acutes			Chronics		
	N	Mean	S.D.	N	Mean	S.D.	N	Mean	S.L.
Education	95	2.49	.33	124	2.37	.46	500	2.26	.33
Job	95	2.72	.22	124	2.40	.43	500	2.25	.36
Housekeeping	95	2.70	.49	118	2.73	.53	466	2.67	.60
Welfare	95	2.77	.53	124	2.61	.64	500	2.11	.81
Finances	95	2.55	.45	124	2.56	.60	498	2.42	.66
Living circumstances	43	1.81	.78	60	1.53	.64	278	1.50	.66
Parents	95	2.73	.33	123	2.60	.64	489	2.46	.47
Relatives	90	2.65	.31	117	2.60	.39	457	2.48	.54
Marriage	71	2.65	.33	51	2.43	.41	249	2.24	.50
Children	45	2.56	.54	38	1.95	.38	175	1.96	.74
Dating	53	2.51	.48	105	2.12	.71	442	1.92	.56
Sex	95	2.74	.42	124	2.35	.53	499	2.24	.76
Friends	95	2.66	.23	124	2.52	.72	500	2.30	.55
Neighbors	95	1.86	.64	124	1.87	.47	494	1.67	.66
Others	95	2.50	.43	124	2.14	.71	500	1.94	.62
Leisure	95	1.85	.70	124	2.17	.56	500	2.08	.34
Religion	95	1.85	.70	124	1.81	.33	500	1.84	.68
Drinking	95	2.73	.38	124	2.59	.68	500	2.59	.61
Addictive drugs	95	2.99	.10	122	2.77	.58	491	2.74	.58
Psychedelic drugs	94	2.72	.67	121	2.49	.53	496	2.63	.75
Antisocial acts	95	2.88	.41	123	2.58	.85	498	2.22	.83
Grand mean	95	2.53	.16	124	2.36	.70	500	2.23	.24

Note: Differences in N are due to the fact that certain items were inappropriate for certain proportion of subjects.

the results show that normals were functioning on a higher level of proficiency than the acutes, and the acutes on a higher level than the pseudoambulatory chronics.

Stress

Table 4−4 presents the means and standard deviations of the D stress scores in the 21 categories of the SSFIPD for the normals and acute and chronic schizophrenics. The grand mean for each group is also presented.

In general, chronic patients showed higher levels of stress than the acutes, who in turn showed greater stress than the normals. Results pf analyses of variance on the stress scores of 19 categories (reduced to 19 because normals were not taking addictive drugs and did not manifest antisocial behavior) and for the mean of the categories showed the groups to be significantly different on 15 categories (Education, Job, Finances, Living Circumstances, Parents, Relatives, Marriage, Children, Dating, Sex, Friends, Neighbors, Others, Drinking, and Psychedelic Drugs) and on the grand mean of the categories. Table 4−5 presents these results.

When the Scheffé method of comparing means was employed, it was found that chronic patients demonstrated significantly more stress than the acutes on 10 categories (Education, Job, Finances, Living Circumstances, Parents, Relatives, Marriage, Dating, Friends, Others) and more stress than normals on 12 categories (Education, Living Circumstances, Parents, Relatives, Marriage, Children, Dating, Sex, Friends, Neighbors, Others, Drinking, and Psychedelic Drugs). A comparison of acutes and normals showed that acutes demonstrated significantly more stress on 6 categories (Children, Dating, Neighbors, Others, Drinking, and Psychedelic Drugs). When the grand means of the groups were compared, it was found that chronics showed significantly more stress than both normals and acutes, and acutes showed significantly more stress than normals.

Functioning vs. Stress

In order to determine the relationship between a subject's level of functioning and his level of stress, correlations between D functioning and D stress scores were computed. Pearson correlation coefficients were determined for chronics, acutes, and normal subjects across the 21 categories of the SSFIPD. Table 4−6 presents these correlation coefficients. An examination of Table 4−6 indicates that, in general, functioning and stress were substantively intercorrelated. The normal subjects showed 13 out of 19 categories intercorrelated

Table 4–3. Analysis of Variance: Comparison of D Function Scores for Normals and Acute and Chronic Schizophrenics for 21 Functioning Categories

Category	Among Groups		Between Groups F Values		
	F	df	N vs. Ac	N vs. Ch	Ac vs. Ch
Education	14.85***	2/716	4.91*	26.36***	7.38***
Job	70.41***	2/716	43.10***	136.56***	16.92***
Housekeeping	0.53	2/676	—	—	—
Welfare	45.76***	2/716	2.56	62.94***	44.54***
Finances	3.29*	2/714	0.02	3.14	4.59*
Living circumstances	4.02*	2/378	4.31*	8.02**	0.12
Parents	16.64***	2/704	4.70*	28.88***	9.22**
Relatives	6.52**	2/661	0.61	9.59***	5.73*
Marriage	27.64***	2/368	7.83**	52.61***	9.04**
Children	13.43***	2/255	15.11***	25.80***	0.00
Dating	29.72***	2/597	18.12***	54.44***	10.71**
Sex	18.73***	2/715	15.19***	37.28***	2.29
Friends	25.61***	2/716	4.20*	40.68***	18.76***
Neighbors	6.50*	2/710	0.01	6.53*	8.77**
Others	37.67***	2/716	19.98***	71.75***	11.39***
Leisure	16.38***	2/716	6.25*	29.73***	7.21**
Religion	0.17	2/716	—	—	—
Drinking	2.29	2/716	—	—	—
Addictive drugs	8.77***	2/705	9.08**	17.52***	0.32
Psychedelic drugs	2.66	2/708	—	—	—
Antisocial acts	35.18***	2/713	8.68***	59.67***	21.09***
Grand mean	77.27***	2/716	28.24***	139.31***	35.35***

$* p < .05$ $** p < .01$ $*** p < .001$

(Footnote to Table 4–3)

Description of 21 Functioning Categories (Appendix A)

1. Education contains 16 functioning items covering level of education achieved, ability to successfully complete training programs, past and present performance in school, etc.

2. Job dimension consists of 25 functioning items covering current employment status, reasons for unemployment and job related problems.

3. Housekeeping consists of 4 functioning items related to effective homemaking.

4. Welfare dimension comprises 4 functioning items pertaining to experience with public assistance, its extent and duration.

5. Management of finances consists of 3 functioning items focusing on manner of handling money, and difficulties with their living standard.

6. Living circumstances contains 1 item for functioning referring to efforts toward improvement of living conditions.

7. Relationship with parents is made up of 4 functioning items focusing on the quality of the relationship and the degree of dependency: interferences by parents in patient's life, criticism, lack of support, etc.

8. Relatives dimension covers 3 functioning items referring to the quality of the relationship and degree of dependence on relatives.

9. Marriage dimension consists of 19 functioning items covering past and present marital interaction and quality of current marriage.

10. Relationship with children covers 7 functioning items pertaining to the quality of the relationship and care taking ability.

11. Dating consists of 5 functioning items pertaining to interest in and ability to relate to opposite sex.

12. Sex consists of 11 functioning items focusing on the ability and difficulty in establishing sexual relationships.

13. Social relationships with close friends consists of 12 functioning items concerned with success in making and keeping of friends, the length and quality of these relationships.

14. Social relationships with neighbors contains 3 functioning items covering the extent and quality of contact.

15. Relationship to others consists of 7 functioning items related to uneasiness with others, degree of enjoyment of group activities, and evaluation of treatment received from others including authority.

16. Spare time interest contains 14 functioning items covering the extent of involving such activities as hobbies, entertainment and travel.

17. Religion dimension consists of 1 functioning item covering church attendance and religious beliefs.

18. The drinking dimension consists of 6 functioning items pertaining to the amount and reasons for drinking, and success in stopping; also problems created by drinking in relation to one's job and personal and social life.

19. Addictive drugs consists of 4 functioning items covering the frequency of and reasons for the use of drugs, and success in forsaking their use; also the effect of drug use on work, personal and social life of the user.

20. Psychedelic drugs dimension contained 2 functioning items assessed in the same manner as addictive drugs.

21. Antisocial acts consists of 13 functioning items covering types of law violations and record of arrests; the effects on the patient of these unlawful activities.

Table 4–4.   Means and Standard Deviations of D Stress Scores for Normals and Acute and Chronic Schizophrenics on the 21 Stress Categories

Category	Normal			Acute			Chronic		
	N	Mean	S.D.	N	Mean	S.D.	N	Mean	S.D.
Education	95	2.35	0.47	124	2.29	0.48	500	2.17	0.51
Job	93	2.62	0.22	122	2.65	0.32	499	2.54	0.38
Housekeeping	74	2.62	0.58	73	2.73	0.56	273	2.55	0.71
Welfare	21	2.41	0.60	44	2.56	0.64	315	2.44	0.63
Finances	95	2.35	0.68	124	2.49	0.62	500	2.27	0.71
Living circumstances	95	2.39	0.68	124	2.36	0.76	499	2.14	0.85
Parents	76	2.55	0.46	106	2.43	0.54	416	2.22	0.61
Relatives	90	2.85	0.26	117	2.77	0.41	455	2.66	0.55
Marriage	71	2.50	0.32	51	2.48	0.36	248	2.33	0.41
Children	43	2.60	0.57	40	2.12	0.89	171	2.20	0.86
Dating	53	2.73	0.30	105	2.54	0.39	443	2.43	0.42
Sex	95	2.67	0.57	124	2.56	0.64	500	2.42	0.72
Friends	95	2.72	0.35	124	2.61	0.59	499	2.41	0.69
Neighbors	95	2.81	0.49	123	2.58	0.74	494	2.58	0.74
Others	95	2.49	0.36	124	2.19	0.45	500	2.05	0.51
Leisure	95	2.52	0.50	124	2.66	0.52	500	2.60	0.54
Religion	89	2.87	0.28	122	2.85	0.30	489	2.83	0.29
Drinking	7	2.69	0.23	31	2.22	0.64	148	2.11	0.58
Addictive drugs	1	0.00	0.00	23	1.97	0.71	95	1.98	0.70
Psychedelic drugs	13	2.69	0.46	36	2.00	0.74	127	2.16	0.75
Antisocial acts	8	1.00	0.00	29	1.21	0.25	237	1.22	0.29
Grand mean	95	2.60	0.44	124	2.50	0.55	500	2.36	0.59

Note: Differences in N are due to the fact that certain items were inappropriate for certain proportion of subjects.

significantly, the acutes had 11 out of 21 categories, and the chronic patients 12 out of 21.

With few exceptions, the correlations between functioning and stress for each of the three groups were significant at the .01 level. Since the scoring system for functioning was the inverse of that for stress (the greater the numerical value of the score, the higher the functioning, but the lower the stress), the positive correlation coefficients actually indicate a negative relationship between stress and functioning. Every significant correlation, but one, for all three groups is positive. It can be concluded, therefore, that the higher the level of functioning a subject demonstrates, the lower will be his level of stress. This relationship hold at about the same degree for all three groups of subjects. It should be pointed out that, in most cases, the correlations that reach significance maintain this significance across the three groups, showing a consistency of relationship between stress and functioning within a particular category for normals and schizophrenic patients.

The final results are related to the determination of short term prediction of the 21 functioning categories. In order to determine these factors a stepwise discriminant function analysis was performed, for 114 readmitted and 91 nonreadmitted chronics, and 33 readmitted and 37 nonreadmitted acutes. The stepwise analysis permitted comparison of the groups on the most discriminating variables alone and in increasing combinations with each of the next best discriminators.

The result indicated that readmission in chronic schizophrenics is favored by 5 functioning categories, of which antisocial behavior ($F = 8.07, p < 0.001$), poor interpersonal relationship with the opposite sex ($F = 7.13, p < 0.001$) and neighbors ($F = 6.95, p < 0.01$) play a predominant part. Lack of religious affiliation ($F = 6.25, p < 0.01$) also contributed to readmission. For the acute patient, functioning with parents ($F = 12.43, p < 0.001$) and friends ($F = 10.34, p < 0.001$) appear to be the major factors leading to readmission, followed by inadequate relationship with the opposite sex ($F = 8.25, p < 0.01$) and uncomfortable living conditions ($F = 7.24, p < 0.01$), job ($F = 6.6$), marriage ($F = 6.20$), and neighbors ($F = 5.71$), contributed less significantly ($p < 0.05$) to readmission.

Table 4–5. Analysis of Variance: Comparison of D Stress Scores for Normals and Acute and Chronic Schizophrenics for 21 Stress Categories

Category	Among Groups		Between Groups F Values		
	F	df	N vs. Ac	N vs. Ch	Ac vs. Ch
Education	6.55**	2/716	0.81	9.99**	5.30*
Job	4.83**	2/711	0.36	3.19	7.95*×
Housekeeping	2.13	2/417	—	—	—
Welfare	0.75	2/377	—	—	—
Finances	4.90**	2/716	2.06	1.04	9.56**
Living circumstances	6.57**	2/715	0.10	8.05**	7.44**
Parents	13.71**	2/595	1.88	20.82***	11.14***
Relatives	6.72**	2/659	1.55	11.25***	4.31*
Marriage	7.26***	2/367	0.07	10.73	6.50*
Children	4.72**	2/251	7.03**	8.20**	0.29
Dating	13.81***	2/598	7.71**	24.85***	5.59*
Sex	5.91**	2/716	1.27	9.79**	3.84
Friends	12.27***	2/715	1.51	18.69***	9.93**
Neighbors	4.24*	2/709	5.60*	8.20**	0.00
Others	34.03***	2/716	20.10***	65.71***	8.71**
Leisure	2.14	2/716	—	—	—
Drinking	3.53*	2/183	3.70*	6.56*	0.88
Addictive drugs	—	2/116	—	—	—
Psychedelic drugs	4.26*	2/173	8.50*	6.17*	1.36
Antisocial acts	—	2/271	—	—	—
Grand mean	34.06***	2/716	7.25***	56.34***	22.22***

*** $p < .001$ ** $p < .01$ * $p < .05$

(Footnote to Table 4–5)

Description of 21 Stress Categories
(Appendix B)

1. Education dimension (15 questions) attempts to determine to what extent the subjects were upset by their achieved level of education, especially in comparison to that of their family; their inability to successfully complete a training program; difficulty in following school rules, or worries resulting from inability to continue their education.

2. Job (8 questions) was concerned with stress associated with type of work, unemployment, and problems in obtaining a job.

3. Housekeeping (2 questions) measured the level of upset relating to ineffective homemaking.

4. Welfare (3 questions) dealt mainly with the subjects' worries about being a welfare recipient and the degree to which this affects his personality.

5. Finances (3 questions) rated the degree of subjects' worries associated with income, and living standards.

6. Living circumstances (3 questions) indexed stress associated with lack of comfort, and poor housing conditions.

7. Parent (9 questions) dealt with stressful interactions between the patient and his family in terms of parental interferences in patient's life and work, criticisms, and conflicts over dependency.

8. Relatives (4 questions) scored stress associated with emotional and financial dependency on relatives.

9. Marriage (25 questions) assessed stress associated with present or recent marriage partners in sexual and emotional interactions.

10. Children (3 questions) scored the subjects' level of upset associated with relating to and taking care of children.

11. Dating (4 questions) examined the worries of the patient based on his inability to find, and relate to a member of the opposite sex.

12. Sex (3 questions) dealt with the subjects' upset over inability to establish satisfactory sexual relationships with the opposite sex.

13. Friends (11 questions) measured the worries of the patient about lack of friends, and inability to relate to them on various levels of inter-personal interactions.

14. Neighbors (1 question) scored his experience in relationship to his level of involvement with neighbors.

15. Relationships with people in community (5 questions) indexed social stress experienced by the patient in relation to authority figures and other people with whom he came into contact within the community, as well as the degree of disturbance about inability to participate in community activities.

16. Spare-time (use of leisure, 2 questions) rated the stress placed upon the patient due to his inability to pursue hobbies or other social activity because of lack of funds or fear of socializing.

17. Religion (13 questions) dealt with the subject's feelings of acceptance by the community of his religious beliefs.

18. Drinking (8 questions) scored the stress related to the problems created by drinking in relationship to job, sexual life, family and social life.

19. Addictive drugs (5 questions) rated stress related to the same working, social, and family problems, etc.

20. Psychedelic drugs (2 questions) calculated the stress related to "bad trips" experienced by the subject.

21. Anti-social acts (1 question) dealt with stressful effects on the patient of his anti-social activities which led to his arrest.

Table 4−6. Correlation Between Stress and Functioning for the 21
Categories of the SSFIPD

Category	Normal	Acute	Chronic
Education	.514**	.544**	.433**
Job	.126	.185	.466**
Housekeeping	.470**	.512**	.590**
Welfare	.128	−.060	.011
Finances	.231*	.127	.254**
Living circumstances	−.012	.015	−.015
Parents	.555**	.469**	.432**
Relatives	.405**	.538**	.558**
Marriage	.788**	.742**	.651**
Children	.415**	.373**	.341**
Dating	.331**	.401**	.486**
Sex	.214*	.301**	.216*
Friends	.667**	.655**	.473**
Neighbors	.103	.206*	.112
Others	.238*	.263**	.336**
Leisure	.073	.163	−.004
Religion	.071	.098	−.011
Drinking	−.611**	.069	.112
Addictive drugs	—	−.053	−.048
Psychedelic drugs	.888**	.045	.063
Antisocial acts	—	−.003	.024

** $p < .01$ * $p < .05$

INTERPRETATION

The present study attempts to clarify four important areas related to
the course of schizophrenia in the community, namely (1) the level
of pre-morbid social functioning before hospitalization in acute
schizophrenics; (2) the degree of adaptability to community, between hospitalizations, of the acute and chronic schizophrenics; (3)
the interaction between the level of functioning and stress in schizophrenia as an indicator of the schizophrenics' community living; and
(4) the short term predictive value of the 21 functioning categories
rated for acute and chronic schizophrenics.

The first results of this investigation have the same epidemiological
implications for community psychiatry which support the concept
that the psychosocial onset of schizophrenia is a gradual, progressive
process of emotional and social disorganization beginning years
before the manifested psychoses are evident, as reported previously
by the author (Serban and Woloshin, 1974) and others (Gittelman-
Klein and Klein, 1969; Higgins, 1969).

The present data do not corroborate the conclusions of Birley and
Brown (based on a study of fifty cases) that 50 percent of schizo-

phrenics have an abrupt transition from "normal functioning" to schizophrenia, due to precipitating events in the last three weeks prior to admission. They do not appear to support its corollary that a sudden onset and good premorbid social adjustment are necessarily associated with a favorable prognosis (Langfeldt, 1956; Stephens and Astrup, 1969; Vaillant, 1964). In our study, 44.3 percent of the acute patients, the majority of whom (77.6%) had sudden manifest onset, required multiple hospitalizations within the two-year observation period, and demonstrated a premorbid level of social functioning significantly below that of normals.

The apparent discrepancies between the findings of this study and previous ones appear to be accounted for by the differences in methodological approach. In previous studies, the acute onset was defined only in terms of recent psychological symptomatology, without a specific measurement of the level of functioning for at least six months to one year prior to hospitalization. In our study, the two variables of onset and premorbid functioning were considered simultaneously. In reality, when a true sudden onset is combined with good premorbid adjustment, the diagnosis of schizophrenia may be inappropriate (Gittelman-Klein, and Klein, 1969).

On the other hand, in schizo-affective psychoses the acute symptomatology is typical of schizophrenia, while the course of the illness could shift into one of these three directions: (1) episodic mixture of manic-depressive and schizophrenic symptoms, (2) relapse to full schizophrenia, and (3) change to manic-depressive symptoms and course (Angst, 1966). In our sample, 48.2 percent of the patients with acute schizophrenic episode and 27.3 percent of the schizoaffectives were readmitted. Furthermore, the above-mentioned studies fail to measure comprehensively the levels of subjects' functioning for any adequate period prior to hospitalization, and also fail to compare it to that of normals.

A second conclusion of importance for the community oriented psychiatry refers to the functioning of chronic schizophrenics in the community after their discharge from the hospital. The new community oriented treatment policy is based on the assumption that an early integration of schizophrenics into the social environment will make them more able to sustain the environmental stress under which they have to function. This is based on the assumption that the discharged chronic schizophrenics are able, ready, and interested to readapt to the social organization of the community. Despite all accumulated evidence that the residual thought defect might interfere with acceptance of any psychiatric intervention at the community level, all programs are organized denying these facts. In reality, this thought impairment affects not only the community adjustment efforts of the schizophrenics (by interfering with his interpretation of societal demands), but it prevents him from accepting prolonged therapeutic aftercare upon hospital release.

Firsthand evidence of this situation is suggested by previously published data, which indicate that 70 percent of the schizophrenic patients admitted to this project did not take medication or attend psychiatric services. A closer analysis of these data revealed that, although at discharge the patients indicated a positive attitude towards participation in community programs and continuance of the prescribed medication after release, they did not pursue it. The implication for community psychiatry from these data is overwhelming, suggesting that the general psychiatric practice based on the liberalized concept of voluntary aftercare treatment for schizophrenics is not only invalid scientifically, but detrimental to the patient.

The assumption that the patient accepts and carries out the psychiatrist's recommendations at discharge is fallacious (Serban and Thomas, 1974). Furthermore, the present results suggest that the chronic patients, who become pseudoambulatory by repeated rehospitalizations and discharges, are unable to function in the community and thus experience the highest amount of stress compared with acutes and normals. It is of interest to note that their marginal functioning, which allegedly should reduce the stress to a minimum, is in reality associated with considerable stress. For chronic schizophrenics, as compared with normals, the surrounding world tends to be a source of turmoil; almost everything appears to them to represent either an insurmountable demand which society places on them or unrest induced by frustrating experiences.

It is also interesting to note that the social functioning of the chronic schizophrenics who are reduced to welfare does not diminish their stressful interaction with society. From previously reported data, it appears that they are the first causalities for readmission, independent of attendance at aftercare programs. As reported, it would suggest that welfare, per se, creates a psychological factor which defeats any motivation for self-improvement (Serban and Thomas).

The findings related to short term prediction of outcome are offering insightful data on their impaired functioning, leading to rehospitalization. It was interesting that the reason for rehospitalization of acute schizophrenics was mainly related to difficulty in their adapting to their previous familial or emotional environment. In their transitional stage towards chronicity, the main problems are with the persons on whom they depend emotionally and with whom they are found to be unacceptable. (See Table 4-7.) For the pseudo-ambulatory chronics living together in the community, between hospitalizations, the social performance predictors have lost most of their meaning. Ironically, in regard to the concept of community therapy, the chronics found it difficult to function in the community. This was their main reason for rehospitalization, antisocial behavior, poor sexual relationships, and difficulty in relating to people in welfare or halfway houses. (See Table 4-7.)

These results are not surprising when we take into consideration the attitude of the close relatives who have custody of the patient and do not perceive the needs and stresses affecting the patient. Whatever the course of action the relatives suggest as a positive approach for the integration of the patient into the mainstream of the community is undoubtedly contrary to that perceived by the patient himself. For example, the patients conveyed a negative attitude in their family interactions, or relationships with spouses, friends, or members of the opposite sex. The difference in the attitudes towards the patient's past hospitalizations and his approach to life represent

Table 4-7. Stepwise Discriminant Function Analysis: Comparison of Readmitted and Non-Readmitted Chronic and Acute Schizophrenics on the Best Discriminating Social Functioning Variables

Variables	Readmitted vs. Non-Readmitted Acutes (F value)
Parents (P)	12.43***
Close Friends (CF) + (P)	10.34***
Dating (D) + (P) + (CF)	8.25***
Living Circumstances (LC) + (P) + (CF) + (D)	7.34**
Job (J) + (P) + (CF) + (D) + (LC)	6.66**
Marriage (M) + (P) + (CF) + (LC) + (D) + (J)	6.20**
Neighbors (N) + (P) + (CF) + (LC) + (D) + (J) + (M)	5.71**

Variables	Readmitted vs. Non-Readmitted Chronics (F value)
Antisocial Acts (AA)	8.07***
Sex (S) + (AA)	7.13***
Neighbors (N) + (AA) + (S)	6.95**
Religion (R) + (AA) + (S) + (N)	6.25*
Dating (D) + (AA) + (S) + (N) + (R)	5.66*

*** $p < .001$
** $p < .01$
* $p < .05$

a source of continuous friction between the patient and his family members, resulting in the maladjustment of the patient to the community (Serban et al., 1975).

The third conclusion with important clinical implications brought out by the data is related to the existent interaction between functioning and stress—which is demonstrable in schizophrenics as well as in normals. Significant correlations between functioning and stress are present in ten categories related to the areas of social performance (education, housekeeping); family interaction (parents, relatives, marital partners, and children); and social interpersonal interaction (dating, sex, friends, people in the community). It is interesting to note that only normals show a high correlation between stress and functioning in the area of drinking and drugs, indicating the extent to which they feel affected by the ill effects of alcohol and psychedelics in their daily functioning. The acutes and chronics, who have a higher anxiety than normals and function at a lower level, are not affected in the same manner by alcohol and drugs, since alcohol temporarily reduces their anxiety levels.

It should be noted as well that the normals, acutes, and chronics maintain a particular pattern of interaction between functioning and stress; namely, the levels of functioning and stress are moving in opposite directions. For instance, normals have the highest levels of functioning and lowest amount of stress; acutes have an intermediate level of functioning related to an intermediate amount of stress; while chronics, at the other extreme, have the lowest level of functioning with the highest amount of stress in the continuum from normality to schizophrenic chronicity.

The implications of the present findings are extremely important clinically for the treatment of schizophrenia in the community. It appears that pseudoambulatory schizophrenics are unable to benefit from present community programs, which are not alleviating the stress induced by the patient's community milieu. The assumption that public assistance or a life free of responsibility in the community would create a nonstressful and protective environment, preventing hospitalization, appears to be erroneous. His life in the community appears to be decided by many interacting variables which sometime appear to act alone or in conjunction with others at another time. They can be reduced to two sets of factors. His one set refers to attitudes and compliance with psychiatric recommendations for medication and attendance at aftercare treatment programs, while another set deals with his poor family and societal interaction, with his genetic predisposition representing the response background for all environmental demands (Serban 1975).

In this light, I believe that the effectiveness of community-based intervention programs for the rehabilitation of chronic schizophrenics requires reevaluation on a more objective assessment basis. The emphasis should be directed towards a better measurement of community experienced stress and adequate control of it by innovative programs that can respond to the needs of the patient. The therapy of the schizophrenic should focus on maintenance of his operational adjustment defined by his ability to tolerate stress while he fulfills a productive role in the community. However, one of the most realistic difficulties in approaching this task is created by our own misconception of the patient's ability to decide, on his own, his right for treatment, while his thinking appears to be impaired in this direction.

The assumption that after discharge the patient is aware of his condition and motivated to take steps to ameliorate it, without any compulsory control is one of the main obstacles in the proper implementation of any community mental health program regardless of how beneficial it might be. (Serban and Gidynski 1975). The schizophrenics' residual mental impairment exacerbated by the stresses of living in the community, if not counteracted by controlled attendance at community programs, adds to the continuation of the familiar pattern of repeated hospitalization often preceded by the harmful societal effect of antisocial acts (42.7% of chronics in Bellevue were admitted because of antisocial behavior).

The "right" to stay mentally ill appears to be one of the controversial guarantees of the law of our permissive culture, and it looms in the background of our delivery of mental health services, making our task somewhat Sisyphean.

Discussant I:
Comment and Caveat

William T. Carpenter, Jr.

KLERMAN

Dr. Klerman has presented an important overview which fairly reflects the status of community or outpatient centered care of schizophrenic patients. His paper is carefully balanced and provides an opportunity to emphasize and extend his discussion rather than to present alternative views.

The first point to discuss is Dr. Klerman's critique of the nature of the evidence regarding efficacy of community treatment. He concludes that there is little research data which can be said to bear on this question. This is surely correct. However, maintenance neuroleptic therapy is often thought to be an exception. This is critical, since the availability of antipsychotic drugs has apparently been an essential ingredient in treating schizophrenic patients outside the hospital. While community-based treatment concepts were derived primarily from sociopsychological considerations, many believe the feasibility of community treatment of schizophrenia is based on neuroleptic maintenance.

How adequate, then, is our information regarding the efficacy of neuroleptic therapy in schizophrenic patients. Two recent reviews [1, 2] have appeared documenting the therapeutic effectiveness of maintenance neuroleptic treatment, but these articles also illustrate the limitations of studies to date. Virtually all these studies rely solely on some measure of rehospitalization and/or symptom relapse to represent course and outcome in schizophrenia. Symptom and hospital status are obviously important in the course of a schizophrenic illness, but they hardly represent a comprehensive assessment of the patient's fate.

In the first place, we know that many variables, other than degree of illness, contribute to rehospitalizing a patient. A medically oriented, intact family may be quick to bring a patient to the hospital with mild symptom exacerbation, while an isolated patient may deteriorate severely without coming to medical attention. More important is the discordance found among various aspects of outcome functioning.

Dr. Strauss and I have shown that the extent of hospitalization during a followup period is only modestly related to other areas of functioning, such as work and social competence [3, 4]. Furthermore, the association between any one of these measures at two-year followup and the other measures at five-year followup is minimal, and in some cases negligible [4]. For example, assessing hospital status during a two-year followup gives minimal information about social or work function at five-year followup. Schwartz et al. [5] found discordance among four outcome measures: mental status, social and role functioning, rehospitalization, and consumer satisfaction.

The paucity of long range followup studies further restricts our understanding of pharmacologic treatment effect. Most reports focus on change during hospital stay or brief followup periods, and few studies extend beyond two years. Engelhart [6] has called attention to the diminishing differences between drug and placebo treated patients, as course is followed over a longer period of time. This does not lessen the importance of short term drug effects, but does suggest that we know very little about their comparative long term advantages. Studies assessing the relationship of treatment to outcome are severely limited unless based on multiple outcome dimensions measured over extension periods of time, a point we have discussed more fully elsewhere [7].

This critique should not distract from the important role of psychopharmacology in schizophrenia, but is intended as a reminder that our informational base on pharmacologic therapy, while more developed than that with other treatment modalities, urgently needs expansion with more sophisticated clinical methodology. At this point we can say that neuroleptic medication: (a) effectively reduces flagrant symptomatology in many patients; (b) appears to have a more generalized antipsychotic effect, which often makes brief hospitalization and return to the community feasible; and (c) reduces rehospitalization rates for at least two years post-discharge.

Dr. Klerman indicated that treatment requirements in subgroups of schizophrenia may differ. Since the use of neuroleptic medication in schizophrenia is almost ubiquitous, identification of subgroups who have limited need for pharmacotherapy is important. Two such subgroups are suggested both by the Davis review [1] and a report by Gardos and Cole [8]. While not well characterized as yet, there would appear to be a subgroup drawn from good premorbid, acute onset, first or second psychotic episode patients who respond well to treatment without medication. These patients may actually do better without medication [7, 9], and should not be placed on long term neuroleptic maintenance. A second subgroup is drawn from a more chronic population who show no adverse reaction to withdrawal from medication or are not responding well to begin with [1, 8].

Gardos and Cole have estimated that as many as 50 percent of medicated chronic patients would do as well off drugs [8]. Even if this estimate is high, one can readily justify drug holidays in chronic schizophrenic patients. Interest in these two subgroups is consistent with Leff and Wing's conclusion that drugs play an important role only in the middle prognostic range [10]. That is, good prognostic patients do well no matter what treatment, and the worst prognostic group do poorly regardless. In any case, the risk of developing tardive dyskinesia is substantial in long term neuroleptic treatment—a situation likely to worsen as psychiatrists rely more on depot intramuscular preparations, hence preventing the spontaneous drug holidays brought about by patient noncompliance. Further research directed towards identifying appropriate treatment for various subgroups is a matter of high priority.

A third point made by Dr. Klerman is that hospitalization can be too brief. I fully concur. A trend toward brief hospitalization puts enormous pressure on clinicians to rapidly use medication in an attempt to reduce symptomatology and render the patient sufficiently manageable to permit discharge. This practice compromises several key clinical tasks involved in hospital treatment. The first is diagnosis. Klein [11] has pointed out that pharmacological decisions are frequently made in advance of adequate diagnosis. These hastily made decisions are in response to particular behavioral manifestations that may not be diagnostically discriminating. Hence, the clinician may not choose the proper category of drug; and, once having instituted drug treatment, it is difficult to shift the therapeutic focus unless there is no demonstrable clinical improvement.

Observed improvement tends to reinforce the treatment regimen. Using improvement as a criteria for continuing treatment is a problem since many patients would improve on placebo, and many non-schizophrenic patients show improvement to neuroleptic drugs. For example, a manic patient presenting a confusing diagnostic picture would probably respond to neuroleptic medication, and might be continued on maintenance neuroleptics if the proper diagnosis were never made. Furthermore, if neuroleptic medication is central to treatment early in the hospital course, it is unlikely that proper eval uation of social and work functioning can be done. In many instances it seems to me that we are not treating the patient or even his illness, but rather our truncated clinical vision becomes focused on symptoms which may be chimeric manifestations on multiple underlying processes.

Brief hospitalization may also preclude establishing a strong collaborative relationship for after care. The high dropout rate of patients after leaving the hospital is a major concern for the community treatment of schizophrenia. This short discussion of potential shortcomings of psychopharmacologic treatment and brief hospitalization does not include comment on the more positive goals of psychosocial treatment that might be implemented given sufficient time and interest.

Dr. Klerman mentioned the inadequate social status of many chronic schizophrenic patients found in the community. This point has received far too little attention. The literature is replete with studies which encourage the assumption that being out of the hospital is somehow equivalent to good health. Lamb and Grotzel long ago reported on the plight of many chronic patients who were successfully kept out of hospitals [12]. The vegetated existence described in these patients, should remind us of how woefully inadequate present treatment methods are for many of our schizophrenic patients.

Dr. Klerman also discussed the need for technologic developments in the treatment of schizophrenia. Our field is looking almost exclusively to the pharmacologist, biochemist, and geneticist for future breakthroughs. Our interest in these areas is abundantly justified, but the exclusive attention to biologic factors in the treatment of schizophrenia is unwarranted. Methodologies appropriate to the investigation of psychosocial treatment techniques need to be developed and systematic studies conducted. There are general social factors that interact negatively with schizophrenia. The best example is the social class which has been found to be an important factor in the prevalence of schizophrenia [13] and in the course of the disease [5]. Indeed, despite important progress in some areas of investigation, we do not appear to be on the verge of any major breakthrough of etiologic or therapeutic significance.

SERBAN

Discussing Dr. Serban's paper provides a difficult task for he has reported a study in a cohort of schizophrenic patients, and has explored the relationship between functioning, stress, and course of illness. The strengths of the study are readily apparent. Dr. Serban has studied a large number of patients, he has provided understandable descriptions of acute and chronic schizophrenia, and his study represents a predominantly lower class and urban patient group—a patient group as typical and problematic as one could hope to cope with. He has used a followup period to revise diagnosis when the original clinical picture could be better accounted for by some other illness. This has enabled him to investigate a more homogeneous study group, and he has not used outcome per se as a criteria for revising the diagnosis. Dr. Serban assessed areas of functioning beyond symptomatology and hospital status. Indeed, he attempted to assess the patient's outcome in terms relevant to everyday life.

Dr. Serban found that onset of schizophrenia was gradual and progressive in acute as well as chronic patients. If he is correct, this would require that we revise our current ideas regarding the prognostic significance of an insidious onset. Our studies of prognostic factors [14] also failed to find rapid onset and participating factors to be prognostically significant. However, we had not achieved satisfactory reliability in estimating these events so that failure to be predictive may have been based on poor reliability. In this regard psychometric evaluation of Dr. Serban's instruments is critical.

Dr. Serban found critically impaired function in a large number of his chronic schizophrenic patients. The extent of illness did not, however, preclude the patients experiencing distress over their functional impairment. This is important to note since all too often chronic schizophrenic patients have been unwittingly regarded as something less than human, and their feelings of distress often regarded as symptoms to be eradicated, rather than a meaningful reflection of their inner experience.

There are two important conceptual issues relevant to Dr. Serban's report. The first is whether community stress and functioning impairment are separate variables. I do not believe that the hypothesis that community or environmental stress increased functional impairment was tested in the study. As I understand his methods, Dr. Serban simultaneously assessed the degree of functioning impairment and the patients' *distress* about the impairment (rather than stress leading to the impairment).

The treatment implications of the two concepts are quite different. If a stressful environment increases functional impairment, it would be reasonable to direct treatment towards a reduction of stress. However, if distress over impaired function is being measured, primary treatment might better be directed toward reducing the impairment, on the assumption that the distress will be automatically relieved as function improves. My personal bias is that low expectations and protective environments may be necessary for some patients, but are unwarranted and detrimental to the population of schizophrenic patients as a whole.

Dr. Serban criticized the "liberalized" concept of voluntary aftercare, a concept he regards as scientifically invalid. I agree with him that ordinary aftercare programs fall far short of their goals as effective treatment centers. However, the concept of compulsory treatment requires ethical, moral, and political consideration. It is not a scientific concept subject to validation. The scientific base for our treatment programs is only indirectly related to decisions as to the circumstances under which our society should deprive individuals of their liberties.

CAVEAT

I will close this discussion with a caveat. Those interested in community treatment programs should take note of the difficulties being encountered by psychotherapeutically interested clinicians. Failure to develop appropriate treatment evaluation techniques has resulted in a paucity of data relevant to a critical appraisal of therapeutic efficacy.

As the pendulum swings from psychodynamic towards psychobiology, psychological treatments for schizophrenia are threatened with inadequate support, if not extinction. This does not simply represent our field turning away from treatment approaches which have been shown ineffective; rather it reflects a discontent with the absence of critical evaluation. Likewise, the community psychiatry movement has apparently reached the point where further growth and development will be curtailed in the absence of meaningful assessment of efficacy. Program development can ride the crest of public and professional interest, but it cannot (and probably should not) be sustained indefinitely in the absence of persuasive scientific justification.

Discussant II: Community Care
Is Not "Deinstitutionalization"

Ernest M. Gruenberg

COMMUNITY PSYCHIATRY

"Community psychiatry" is a difficult rubric to discuss from a scientific point of view because the term is used to refer to too many ideas and activities at once. Actually, it is only a fashionable term, used to emphasize the nonhospital aspects of psychiatric work. It refers to a large expansion of what were once called "extramural" programs when organized by mental hospital psychiatrists. It also refers to psychiatric services organized by local agencies, both voluntary agencies and local governments, and in that context, refers to both inpatient and outpatient services. These have expanded phenomenally since World War II. Most of this expansion of community-based services has reflected a tendency for psychiatry to become involved in treatment of people with less severe forms of mental disorders than those to which the government mental hospitals and private mental hospitals catered.

The locally organized psychiatric services which expanded rapidly following New York State's legislative initiative (The Community Mental Health Services Act of 1954 [11]) were of little relevance to the patients who were being cared for in state mental hospitals. Following the development of federally funded Community Mental Health Centers in 1963 [3] there was also little interest in the patients with severe chronic mental disorders. These locally operated services often competed for staff successfully, but the local services rarely competed for patients, and often refused services to people who had been in a mental hospital or seemed likely to need hospitalization soon.

257

COMMUNITY CARE

However, some government mental hospitals developed a pattern of community care for their chronically ill patients that did not depend on local initiatives [8]. Keeping people with severe chronic mental disorders in community placements during prolonged periods of treatment was an important accomplishment. It became linked to a pattern of open hospital care, a system of flexible staff involvement in caring for patients, both while in hospital, and when at home, that clinicians found more interesting and rewarding.

Leighton was right to point out, however, that neither community care nor locally operated clinical services are inherently more virtuous or better than state operated services or hospital services. We should never forget that Horace Mann, Dorothea Dix, and all the founders of the American Psychiatric Association found community care and community services to be so horrible that they persuaded the states to deprive local governments of authority to offer care to the poor mentally ill.

If community care is better for people with severe chronic mental disorders, it is because it prevents severe chronic deterioration. The *benefit* of this new technology is that it prevents chronic deterioration in personal and social functioning.

CHRONIC DETERIORATION
TO BE PREVENTED

Sometimes people with severe mental disorders develop behavior patterns that destroy their social relationships. There are a limited variety of such behavioral patterns and they have been labelled the "social breakdown syndrome" (SBS). These reactions can be viewed as following one of three patterns: (a) withdrawal, (b) anger and hostility, (c) combinations of these two.

Withdrawal is manifested by loss of interest in the surrounding world, sometimes accompanied by intense preoccupation with an inner phantasy life. As patients withdraw in this way they lose interest in social functions such as work responsibilities, housekeeping functions, and ordinary social obligations. Interest in personal appearance, dress, bodily cleanliness, and toilet also decline. In the end comes the standard picture of the deteriorated, dilapidated, unresponsive, soiling, helpless, vegetative creature who in former times inhabited our mental hospitals' back wards.

The pattern of anger and hostility is manifested by expressions of resentfulness, quarrelsomeness, and hostility. When more advanced along this path the patient may accuse others of intent to harm him and become physically aggressive and assaultive. He may turn his wrath upon physical objects and become destructive of windows, furniture, or household fixtures; or his wrath may become directed at himself and this may lead to self-mutilating activities or outright suicide.

In those instances where the pattern pursued mixes tendencies to withdraw and tendencies toward hostility and anger, combinations of the features of both paths may appear. In addition, there is a way of withdrawing aggressively by distortions of the usual responsiveness to other people, for example, by stubbornly echoing whatever anyone else says, by assuming bizarre poses of body position or speech patterns, by odd gesticulations, and so forth. These modes of response avoid the "nonresponsiveness" of pure withdrawal and the overt expressions of resentment such as cursing and striking out, while effectively preventing real personal contact and indirectly expressing resentment or enmity.

These pathways toward destruction of an individual's social relations have long been observed and described [1].

The limited number of behaviors in the SBS which occur in a wide variety of mental disorders, makes this syndrome similar to Selye's "general adaptation syndrome"; the general adaptation syndrome refers to the organism's inability to maintain the stability of the "milieu intérieur." while SBS describes decompensations in the individual's integration into the social milieu.

Community care practices preserve the patients' sense of self-respect and feeling of responsibility for their own behavior. Here are some of the principles by which it works:

1. Eliminate locks and other physical restraints.
2. Release as soon as the admission-related crisis is past. Such early release requires easy readmission whenever the clinical, personal or family situation demands it. If timely readmissions are resisted, rejecting attitudes toward difficult patients will develop early, and community placements will become difficult or impossible [10].
3. Half the hospital staff's case load is in the community where the staff does followup and is continuously available for consultation with patient, family and community physicians, nurses, social workers, and police.
4. A community care service can serve only a small area. Short channels of communication and familiarity with local community resources and personnel are needed. A big staff for a big area does not work.

What distinguishes a service devoted to providing community care for long term seriously handicapped mental patients is the existence of a clinical team which can provide both inpatient and outpatient services as the patients' needs change from time to time. Such a team can be called a "unified clinical team" since it continues to take responsibility for a set of patients when they move from inpatient to outpatient to day hospital or other "transitional" forms of care [6].

Community Care Preceded CPZ

Community care was already operating in some communities when the first tranquilizing drug became widely known in 1953. For example, Duncan Macmillan said in 1957:

> We began in 1945 and we completed it in 1952. . . . We have reduced our numbers by over 300 since 1949. In 1949 we had over 1,300 beds in the hospital, and now we have just about 1,000. . . .
> It might be of interest to mention that I carried out a review of all the first admissions to the hospital during the year 1954, that is, all those who were first admitted during the year, in order to find out how many were still in the hospital. I found that only eleven were still in the hospital. Of these, six are senile cases and one is a child in the children's unit. Not one is a case of schizophrenia. So the community is now locally playing a large part in the rehabilitation of the patient. There were 1,196 admissions in that year altogether, first admissions and readmissions combined [10].

The United States began to import community care from Britain and new drugs from France in the years following 1955. Because tranquilizing drugs make community care easier, some assumed that community care was caused by tranquilizing drugs.

Chronic SBS Can Be Prevented

In January 1960 psychiatric services (excluding those for alcoholism and mental retardation) for residents aged 16−65 of Dutchess County, New York were reorganized to provide the type of unified community care program described above. Because the major goal of the Dutchess County demonstration was to reduce the incidence of chronic SBS, a research unit was established to evaluate the impact of the new services. Figure 4−1 shows the decrease in episodes of chronic SBS after initiation of the services. The unified community care program reduced the annual frequency of episodes of chronic SBS from over 40 per 100,000 general population to less than 16 per 100,000. Since the condition lasts many years, at least 75 person-years of severe disability are saved each year for each 100,000 population getting a unified community care service [7].

The introduction of community care also reduced the number of hospital beds occupied by about 50 percent in ten years. This drop

Figure 4–1. Estimated Number of Episodes of Chronic Social Breakdown Syndrome Beginning Each Year in Persons Aged 16–65 in Dutchess County, New York. Area between curves measures person-years of chronic SBS prevented by community care. (From reference 7)

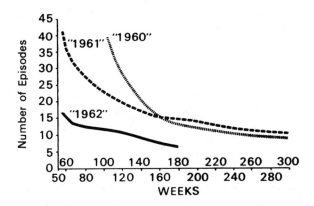

occurred despite rising first admissions and readmissions because the length of stay following admission dropped even more dramatically. Since 1965, in Dutchess County, New York, half of all admissions have been released within two weeks.

Easy Release Requires Ready Readmissions

"Deinstitutionalization" is a slogan which confuses issues. Institutional censuses did drop with community care programs because the "easy-out" practice shortened hospital stays even faster than the complementary "easy-in" practice raised admission and readmission rates. Hence, a hospital census drop with rising readmission rates became an *indicator* of a service system moving toward a good pattern of community care. To call a policy "deinstitutionalization" substitutes this indicator for the desired phenomenon—something like a child trying to push the speedometer needle to make a car go faster.

Why do so many who wish to seize on a part manifestation to represent the whole, seize on dropping census rates instead of on rising readmission rates? Both are equally good indicators of progressive policies. Is it to impress budget directors? Or is it to enhance our self-image as effective therapists? "Deinstitutionalization" also encourages the notion that all chronic deterioration (or chronic SBS) is a *product* of institutional life. Institutional neurosis, as described by Russel Barton, occurs [2]. However, many cases of chronic SBS are well established before hospitalization.

ALL DETERIORATION IS NOT INSTITUTIONALISM

In 1963 our research unit reviewed the 50 cases of chronic SBS existing in Dutchess County who had become deteriorated after the community care pattern began in January 1960 [12]. Half of these cases were schizophrenic, 19 were organic brain syndromes, and 10 were other functional disorders, indicating that any psychiatric disorder can provide a fertile ground for secondary sociogenic disabilities.

Table 4–8, which shows the distribution of these 50 cases by locus of onset and behavior pattern, reveals that 17 episodes of deterioration had begun prior to hospitalization, while 33 originated in an institutional setting. Most of the institution onsets (25 of the 33) fit Barton's description of institutional neurosis, but eight of them, and all of the community onsets, showed no institutional neurosis symptoms. These data suggest that only about half of the episodes of chronic deterioration that occur can be explained as a response to an institutional environment. Hence, merely reducing long-term hospital admissions will inevitably leave some cases of secondary disability unaffected. About half of the savings in chronic deterioration which occurred in Dutchess County when good community care programs were introduced were due to a quick termination of social breakdown syndrome episodes which began outside of hospitals. The other half which were prevented were the cases of institutional neurosis produced by over-institutionalization.

Experience has shown that the best way to deal with a patient in the community who is beginning to deteriorate in personal or social functioning is to offer a rapid relevant response, sometimes including a brief period of hospital care [4]. If you watch patients who have been withdrawn or combative for up to three or four months coming

Table 4–8. Distribution of Chronic SBS Cases by Locus of Onset and Behavior Patterns

| | Behavior Patterns | | |
Locus of Onset	One or More Institutional Neurosis Symptoms	No Institutional Neurosis Symptoms	Total
Institution	25	8	33
Community	0	17	17
Total	25	25	50

(From reference 12)

into a good open hospital with sympathetic personnel and appropriate preadmission care, you see that the tension, anxiety, and combativeness often melt with 15 minutes of walking through the door. This is not the universal response, but it is very common. It is not due to drugs, because often these have not yet been administered. In my judgment, it must be due to the dramatic initiation into the sick role and an explanation to patients for their sense of failure in managing their own lives.

REHABILITATING CHRONIC SBS

The discussion so far has emphasized the efficacy of unified clinical services in preventing chronic deterioration. But how effective are such services in rehabilitating already chronic SBS? The only data available on this question indicate that while the services do help some patients, they are less effective in rehabilitating people who have already developed chronic SBS than they are in preventing SBS episodes from becoming chronic [9]. On the basis of surveys repeated every six months up to September 1962, Table 4–9 shows the recovery rates for Dutchess County and non-Dutchess County persons who were on chronic wards in September 1959. The rate of improvement after 1959 is too slow to enable us to anticipate that 100 percent of these chronic SBS patients will become fully rehabilitated. Without a new discovery, it is inevitable that some of these patients will require institutional care for the rest of their lives. Moreover, there is no evidence to suggest that moving them from one kind of institution to another will help them to recover faster.

Table 4–9. Percentage of Continuously Severe SBS Patients Who Were Rated Free of Severe SBS on Each Survey

	Dutchess County		*Non-Dutchess County*	
	n	*%*	*n*	*%*
September 1959	268	36.6	267	36.7
January 1960	165	30.9	168	17.3
September 1960	111	30.6	139	12.4
January 1961	76	11.8	119	8.4
September 1961	67	14.9	107	7.5
January 1962	57	12.3	98	12.2
September 1962	50	4.0	83	20.5

(From reference 9)

CONCLUSION

In this discussion I have presented evidence to show that the goal of preventing chronic SBS is not only possible to achieve but is also the only logical goal for us to pursue if we are sincere in our desire to minimize the burden of chronic deterioration to the individual, community, and society. But we also know that achieving this end is a more complex matter than that conveyed by slogans such as deinstitutionalization. In a sense, a community care program achieves deinstitutionalization by detotalizing the place where inpatient care is provided and by proffering the clinical staff which works on the inpatient services to seriously ill patients who are living outside of the hospital. It blurs the distinction between inpatient and outpatient care by having the same clinical team provide both. This is in contrast to deinstitutionalization which dumps inpatients into communities without providing continuing hospital-based services, which too often ends up as a form of community neglect. It is also in contrast to programs which, in an effort to prevent readmissions (a large number of which are to be expected), create mini-institutions which are even less flexible and stimulating than the parent hospital was or could become; this leads only to fragmented institutionalization [5].

We have learned that if we adopt an attitude of acting on our best hopes, backed up with readiness to act on our worst fears, our patients do less badly than if we permit ourselves to act on our worst fears without giving hope a chance. Pending major advances in technique or knowledge, using intermittent hospitalization flexibly is the most effective way we have for making the best out of what is—if we are to be truthful with ourselves—a very poor job.

Closing Remarks:
A Critical Appraisal

Lawrence C. Kolb

The theme of this symposium of the Kittay Scientific Foundation undoubtedly received much of its impetus from the evident critical appraisal of the community mental health movement, as its weaknesses have become so publicly conspicuous and so controversial in the world's most complex social environment—that is, the megalopolis of New York.

In this environment one must contend with the value systems of a multitude of ethnic groups—highly divergent socioeconomic status among its population (although these are much less conspicuous than evident in many other nations),—and a health delivery system so complicated and so devoted in its individual components to the integrity of local territorial power, that it is no wonder the representatives of the consumers have created a furor over the evident human expressions of failure in the movement.

Dr. Yolles emphasized the primary goal of the Community Mental Health Act of 1963 as directed to offsetting the deleterious effect of chronic long term institutional care through the establishment of many local centers providing early diagnosis, treatment, and the hopeful retention within the local community for care of the majority of those with mental and emotional illness. This goal is indeed one with which everyone in this audience will agree. He suggested that if the planning were to be redone today it is likely that the legislative act would be similar to the one shaped and made a federal statute in 1963. I wonder! The act, as well as New York's original Community Mental Health Act, its present Unified Services Act, as well as the new federal PL 94–63, to my mind have a similar flaw—the failure to define clearly governance, and establish effective interrelationships between different segments of the delivery system.

As Mitchell Gordon wrote many years ago in *Sick Cities* (where 70 percent of the U.S. population now lives), ''The mosaic of local authorities in a single metropolitan area results in increasingly wasteful duplications of local services, conflict and confusion in their execution, inequities in taxation and, in many instances, complete paralysis in the solution of more and more urgent areawide needs.''

There has been a tendency in this country to believe that, by adding another newer layer of bureaucracy supported with funds and a new goal, problems will be solved. If we were to truly plan for the future (or to rethink the past), perhaps the interrelationship between institutional structures and delivery of mental health services would be more effectively outlined and incentives given so that any new structure clearly relates to the pre-existing structures and those foreseen in the future.

The weaknesses exposed in the community mental health movement in the large cities or suburban areas where most of our people now live, derive in considerable part from the planning processes which overlooked organizational interrelations and took little cognizance of potential negative local attitudes towards living with supporting the rehabilitation of the mentally ill. It also overlooked incentives to administrators to achieve the stated goals and penalties for them in deviating from those same goals.

Yet the movement has been a success for the most part. Personally, I doubt that it would have taken place without the new therapeutic developments, particularly those in psychopharmacology, to the changing attitudes toward the mentally ill, and without the development of a vast cadre of supportive persons (professionals and nonprofessionals) encouraged and eager to provide the necessary therapeutic interventions. It is a success—, in spite of the conspicuous social incompetence of many of the previously institutionalized, now attracting attention in a variety of communities, urban, suburban, and rural.

It is not generally known that in New York State today, 65 percent of those seriously disturbed and admitted to the state facilities from the front line services return to their own family and marital homes when discharged. The remainder are housed in a variety of residential settings. It might be worth mentioning that only 2 percent are in SROs (single room occupancies) in the metropolitan area.

In the light of Dr. Srole's paper, it is of interest to note that some 2,500 families throughout this state alone offer care to approximately 7,800 persons with various forms of mental disability. The majority of those so treated live in rural communities, but now major efforts are underway to place in family care, particularly, the re- tarded, in this vast metropolitan area. Dr. Srole pointed up the value of concentration of family care as it exists in Geel. Yet the attitudes of Geel and its people were shaped over centuries. We must study the effects of density of concentration of social deviance.

Bruce Dohrenwend quoted Caplan who stated the goal of the com- munity mental health movement as dedication to the reduction of the incidence of mental illness. This ambitious goal, (if Caplan meant reduction through the means of primary prevention), has undoubt- edly been completely missed. The achievement of this goal was ex- pected in that vast social experiment made in the USSR through its revolution. It is unfortunate that the invited guests to this conference from that country were unable to attend, as the Russian psychiatrists now freely confess that this massive social experiment as related, in which the expectation was held of reduction of incidence of the major psychoses, has been a failure. They yearn to prove that per- haps they have limited the neurotic processes. Certainly drug abuses, in the form of alcoholism and psychopathy, abound in that and other socialist countries, suggesting that the major etiologic forces for these conditions antedate the influence of social conditioning and exist in the transactions between biological and familial forces.

I found Alec Leighton's analysis of the frequencies of disorder in the small community he studied of enormous interest, particularly since he emphasized the large proportion (almost 75 percent) who were in need of medical care and the fact that, in spite of community educational efforts after fifteen years, the vast proportion continued to be referred to the mental health subsystem as entrants from the health system per se. This fact deserves emphasis particularly among our legislators, both federal and state, many of whom have been "conned" into believing that physician-psychiatrists may be replaced by either family physicians, other mental health professionals or non- professionals.

The failure to sustain the medical component in the mental health manpower series through direct subsidization in the years ahead may be foreseen as perhaps an initial regression toward the institutional model of care, unless the country develops and licenses special health personnel able and privileged to provide much of the work now done by psychiatrists. Dr. Leighton advised me informally (after my com- ments on the potential existence of social homeostasis, and its pos- sible disruption by too much deviance or variability of levels of tension acceptable to allow community competence), of relevant studies related to this hypothesis done in this area some 30 years ago.

To me, both the conclusions and recommendations made by Professors Dohrenwend and Langner provided us with guidelines as well as delimitations of our capacities as professionals in urging social change and experimentation as a prevention of psychosocial disabilities. It would indeed be interesting to carry out on a small scale the development of a Utopian poverty-free group to retest the hypothesis that socioeconomic factors are major forces in producing personality disorder. I have already mentioned the failure to so demonstrate that relationship in the USSR, but perhaps in another less repressive society, the hopes of modifying the occurrence of the neuroses and personality disorders might be achieved.

Personally, I would bet against modifying the incidence of psychoses over time in the course of such a social experiment. Langner's analysis of the strong factors found to relate to behavioral disorders in childhood suggests the possible value of alleviation of social and family stress, in reduction or prevention of childhood disorder. But, in fact, is it possible to modify pre-existing intrapsychic parental pathology of parents by simple social engineering? We do not know. Yet, very probably, the shift in such pathology would occur only after some generations of less stressful environmental life.

For the pragmatic approach to our current problems of managing more effectively the successful assessment of community attitudes and the potential for supportive aid to the relocated mental patient in communities, Dr. Struening's discussion on social area analysis resounded as a most encouraging lead. We must know much more of the social area and social network characteristics in planning continued treatment in the various communities, and employ that knowledge effectively in the field, if we are to escape the currently damaging criticism given the mental health providers. However, will social area analysis detect well the potential energetic paranoid leader with strongly aversive attitudes towards the mentally disabled? Dr. Tischler demonstrated this approach in his report in terms of a selection of service, with his comment that certain areas submit to the continued exposé of annual institutional readmission rates of 66−2/3 percent.

In New York State, we have commenced an analytic study of the pressing issue of readmission. But will it be possible, in the light of the legal constraints now placed upon those working in the field, to modify the practice of easy discharge into the community, so as to escape the necessity of waging battles in the courts? As a perceptive social worker has reported to me, the institutional psychiatrists have simply given up and are awaiting a public reaction formation against those eagerly pushing the civil rights demands of those admitted to the hospital. There are few psychiatrists today who will insist on fighting for retention in order to treat, in spite of the verbiage about rights to treatment.

Glick's fine study provides the potential for clinical decision making as related to various defined groups. I found myself interested in his findings that the "poor premorbids" do just as well or better with either short or long term hospitalization. In that country, where community psychiatry has existed for many years, and where its emergence was forced on the society due to lack of housing (the USSR), there were many reports given during last year's international symposium on social rehabilitation, which Dr. Cancro and I had the pleasure of attending, as the representatives of this country. I noted particularly the open reporting of incapacity to effect useful social rehabilitation in about one-third of the cases.

A most revealing informal bit of information given me there is the fact that there is no organized series of statutes dealing with the mentally ill in Russian law. Shostakovitch (the nephew of the great composer) is pressing for such statutes. He advised me that only one law existed on the books, and that allows the individual identified as a mental patient (usually a psychotic) to have a full room of individual living space—a privilege not allowed to the general public. I assume the Russian public, not unlike most of the western public, has found a certain degree of space distancing necessary in their daily transactions with the psychotic, in order to sustain the general mental health.

Tishler's findings that greatest changes effected by treatment occurred in personal adjustment factors and less in role skills serve to point up the problems of current interventions to assist the mentally ill. At the press conference I emphasized the need for improved personality theory, which would define positive sets conducive to social competence. As Dr. Leighton commented, some work has emerged in this area, but to me the specificity contained in the use of such concepts of "mental health" or "coping" are insufficient to guide therapeutic learning techniques to bring about effective change, leading to positive balance in personality and thus social competence.

A good deal of my reflective time in the past several years has been given to thinking on this subject. Empirically, it occurs to me that the behavioral techniques now used in the schools for the retarded do indeed provide learning experiences which establish assets necessary to adapt well socially. But the problem of establishing social competence is vastly more complex when concerned with our major problem—the schizophrenic—where pathology inhibits or deters the use of social skills, even if once learned.

With these thoughts in mind, as administrator, I have restated the goal of our state department as one that must go beyond the relief of distress due to psychopathology to that of social rehabilitation. Serban's work points up the necessity of interventions which accomplish such competence before placing the long term chronic schizophrenics. I would suggest that only by establishing within the individual the skills that make one socially competent, will those suffering be relieved of the additional stress many of them find living in the community. Serban's findings also mandate the necessity for effective after care—reaching out to the formerly institutionalized, to assure their necessary medical and psychosocial continuing care.

In conclusion, I would address myself briefly to the significance of this conference, particularly in the light of Dr. Mosher's concerns. The state of any professional art improves through critical, or shall I call it scientific, search and research. It is my belief that the contributions of all those who have participated in this symposium will foster the continuance of the community mental health movement.

We have identified here the patient groups towards whom greatest attention must be directed—and the schizophrenic clearly needs the most attention. We have promise of more effective analysis of social attitudes to assist us in the selective use of alternative and more stimulating and normative living conditions through the methods of social area analysis here. Thus potentially both stress and need for rehospitalization will be reduced. We have also identified the need for outreach followup for the chronically ill schizophrenic, as well as the necessity for the establishment of stable linkages between provider subsystems to assure the same.

If it is possible within a few years to bring any of the identified needs to operation in the large system with which I am identified, I shall be enormously gratified.

Afterword

RECOMMENDATIONS FOR THE NATIONAL
INSTITUTE OF MENTAL HEALTH

Recommendations were made to the National Institute of Mental Health by the research scientists participating in the fourth international symposium entitled "A Critical Appraisal of Community Psychiatry" sponsored by the Kittay Scientific Foundation. The main issues for recommendation were:

1. The effectiveness of the community mental health center and delivery of services to the community.
2. Evaluation of the program in terms of benefits to the patients.
3. The crucial need for research in this area (community psychiatry).
4. The necessity for a better organized campaign in the Congress or federal government agencies to favor mental health programs.

The Effectiveness of Community
Mental Health Services

In the first area, the recommendations revolved around the need to define the functions of the community mental health center in terms of treatment to patients. It was also emphasized that there existed a need for clarification of the controversy between the medical model and the social one, as a base for the approach to treatment of patients in the community. Dr. Robert Ellsworth suggested that the functioning of the community health center could be improved by monitoring their performance, as related to the true impact of these facilities in the community.

Dr. Louis Jolyon West believes that there is a crying need for clarifying the role of the community health center, in relationship to the appropriate variety of treatment modalities. According to Dr. West, there is a definite need for guidelines regarding the selective use of a particular type of patient regarding treatment.

It was the general consensus that one deficiency of community mental health centers is the inadequate development of programs to ensure continuity of care for various types of community follow-up and treatment (this point was particularly stressed by Dr. Frank Ochberg). At this time, apparently, community mental health care centers are unable to control the patients discharged from hospitals. This, therefore, reinforces state hospitalization as a valid form of institutionalization for the treatment of special categories of patients. (Cancro & Herz).

Dr. Robert Cancro suggested redefining the community mental health center (a misnomer) to community "sick centers," since these centers deal particularly with the treatment of the mentally ill and do not serve to improve the health of the community, which now seems involved with political, social, and economic factors.

Dr. Gary Tischler emphasized the problems of the utilization of the community mental health center in relation to the entitlement to treatment concept. Dr. Tischler proposed a new definition of that concept in order to screen the psychosocial problems which cannot be solved in present community mental health centers.

Evaluation

Suggestions were made in relation to the evaluation program in terms of benefits to patients. The urgency of the problem appears to lie within the context of the status of chronic schizophrenics in the community. Participants were of the opinion that schizophrenics were "dumped" from state hospitals into the community without truly being followed up through rehabilitation programs. Drs. Ernest Gruenberg and George Serban stressed the point that "outside of medication" the chronic patient receives little attention from community programs.

It was also suggested by Dr. Serban that intensive educational programs in the community for families of schizophrenics should be organized, thereby enabling the relatives of these patients to understand the nature of mental illness. He believes that this should be coupled with the creation of innovative care programs which will permit continuance of adequate medical care. He also suggested that mandatory treatment should be initiated for a category of chronic schizophrenic patients with multiple and frequent hospitalizations, who should be then placed in rehabilitative and educational satellite programs associated with a hospital setting for the stabilization of their conditions.

Drs. Heinz Lehmann and Loren Mosher recommended a possible solution which they believe might be appropriate for chronic schizophrenics, through the conversion of certain state hospitals into a "community" of chronic patients, who might then be free to organize their lives on a nonpressurized level.

Dr. Lawrence C. Kolb stressed that the treatment of patients should be clearly defined in terms of various entities of psychopathology and should be related to stages of disturbance. He discussed, in particular, the support service area of the community. Dr. Robert Senescu, along with other participants, recommended that academia should get more involved in the area of community care, in order to improve the quality of service on this level.

Research

It was the general consensus that more longitudinal studies are necessary for evaluating the functioning of mental health centers and for treatment modalities as well. Drs. William Carpenter, Marvin Herz, George Serban, Thomas Langner, Seymour Kety, and Bruce Dohrenwend strongly supported innovative evaluation of treatment for schizophrenics in the community.

Dr. William Carpenter proposed research for identifying the subgroups of schizophrenias, which require different types of treatment from the ones presently available. Dr. Tischler emphasized longitudinal studies of the subject of mental health in order to determine if they produce patients who remain less chronically ill over a period of time, than the treatment presently employed in the state hospitals.

Drs. Dohrenwend, Langner, and Kety expressed their belief that community psychiatry suffers from a paucity of research due to a social enthusiasm which is unsupported by sufficient scientific data. It was mentioned as well that epidemiological studies should be carried out with a normal population sample in order to develop primary prevention approaches to mental illness.

The Role of the Federal Government

It was the general agreement among the participants that the National Institute of Mental Health should conduct a policy of disseminating better information to other governmental agencies and Congress on the significance of more research in the field of mental illness. This will lead to better rehabilitative programs in community psychiatry in order to face the magnitude of the mental health problem which is confronting the nation.

It was the position of several scientists at the meeting (including Drs. Kety, Leighton, Langner, and Dohrenwend) that cancer and cardiac diseases receive a stronger financial support from the government than mental health, due to their lobby and specific nature of the problem, which appear closer to the personal life of people in Congress.

In reply to the general position that insufficient funds are available for the implementation of adequate community mental health networks, Dr. Ochberg explained the budgetary difficulty of the National Institute of Mental Health, in relationship to implementation of sound programs for expanding the necessary research, at the community mental health level. Dr. Ochberg agreed with the need for evaluation of community programs and research for the treatment of chronically ill patients in the community, as a top priority for the improvement of quality in mental health care.

References

FOREWORD

1. Rice, A.K., *Enterprise and Its Environment*, Barnes & Noble, Pennsylvania, 1971.

2. E.J. Miller and A.K. Rice, *Systems of Organization*, Tavistock Publications, New York, 1967.

3. Astrachan, B.M., Levinson, D.J., Adler, D.A., "The Impact of National Health Insurance on the Tasks and Practice of Psychiatry," *Archives of General Psychiatry* 33: 785–794, July 1976.

CHAPTER 1–OCHBERG AND OZARIN

1. Comptroller General of the U.S., *Report to the Congress*, Need for More Effective Management of Community Mental Health Centers Program, B–164031 (S), Aug. 27, 1974.

2. Marmor, J., The Relationship Between Systems Theory and Community Psychiatry, *Hospital and Community Psychiatry*, 26:12 (Dec.) 1975.

3. Thomas, C.S. and Garrison, V., *A General Systems View of Community Mental Health in Progress in Community Mental Health*, Vol. III, edited by Bellak, L. and Barten, H.H., Brunner/Mazel, New York, 1975.

4. Deutsch, A., *The Mentally Ill in America*, Columbia University Press, New York, 1949.

5. Bockhoven, J.S., *Moral Treatment in Community Mental Health*, Springer, New York, 1972.

6. Deutsch, A., *op. cit.*, p. 1505.

7. *Op. cit.*, p. 326.

8. Deutsch, A., *Shame of the States*, Arno Press, New York, 1948.

9. Gorman, M., *Oklahoma Attacks Its Snake Pits*, University of Oklahoma Press, 1948.

10. Greenblatt, M., York, R.H., and Brown, E.L., *From Custodial to Therapeutic Care in Mental Hospitals*, Russell Sage Foundation, New York, 1955.

11. American Psychiatric Association, *Better Care in Mental Hospitals*, Proceedings of the First Mental Hospital Institute, Apr. 11–15, APA, Washington, D.C., 1949.

12. Goffman, E., *Asylums*, Aldine Press, Chicago, 1962.

13. Belknap, I., *Human Problems of a State Mental Hospital*, McGraw-Hill, New York, 1956.

14. Wessen J. (ed.), *The Psychiatric Hospital as a Social System*, C.C. Thomas, Springfield, Ill., 1964.

15. Jones, M., *The Therapeutic Community, a New Treatment Method*, Basic Books, New York, 1953.

16. Jones, M., *Social Psychiatry*, C.C. Thomas, Springfield, Ill., 1962.

17. "European Mental Health Programs as Viewed by Mental Health Specialists and Legislators," Southern Regional Education Board, Atlanta, Ga., (Sept.) 1961.

18. *Mental Hospitals Join the Community*, 39th Annual Conference, Milbank Memorial Fund, New York (Sept.), 1962.

19. Barton, W. et al., *Observations of Psychiatric Practice in Europe*, Mimeographed copy, State of Mass. (undated).

20. *Action for Mental Health*, Final Report of the Joint Commission on Mental Illness and Health, Basic Books, New York, 1961.

21. Greenblatt, M., Moore, R.F., Albert, R.S., and Solomon, M.H., *The Prevention of Hospitalization*, Grune & Stratton, New York, 1963.

22. Glaser, F.B., *The Uses of the Day Program in Progress in Community Mental Health*, Vol. II, edited by Barten, H. & Bellak, L., Grune & Stratton, New York, 1972.

23. Herz, M.I., Endicott, J., and Spitzer, R.L. et al., "Day versus Inpatient Hospitalization, A Controlled Study," *Am. J. of Psychiatry*, 127:1371–1382, 1971.

24. Langsley, D. G., Machotka, P., and Flomenhaft, K., "Avoiding Mental Hospital Admission: A Followup Study," *Amer. J. of Psychiat.* 127:1391–1394, 1971.

25. Dekker, B. and Stubblebine, J., "Crisis Intervention & Prevention of Psychiatric Disability: A Followup Study," *Amer. J. of Psychiat.* 129:6, 725–729, 1972.

26. Glasscote, R.M., Cumming, E., Rutman, I.D., Sussex, J.N., and Glassman, S.M., *Rehabilitating the Mentally Ill in the Community*, A Study of Psycho-Social Rehabilitation Centers, Joint Information Service (APA –NAMH), Washington, D.C., 1971.

27. Fairweather, G.W., Sanders, D.H., Maynard, H., and Cressler, D.L., *Community Life for the Mentally Ill: An Alternative to Institutional Care*, Chicago, Aldine, 1969.

28. Davis, A.E., Dinitz, S., and Pasamanick, B., *Schizophrenics in the New Custodial Community: Five Years After the Experiment*, Ohio State University Press, Columbus, 1974.

29. Michaux, W.W., Katz, M.M., Kurland, A.A., and Gansereit, K.H., *The First Year Out, Mental Patients After Hospitalization*, Johns Hopkins Press, Baltimore, 1969.

30. Mannino, F.V., MacLennan, B.W., and Shore, M.F., *The Practice of Mental Health Consultation*, DHEW Publication (ADM) 74—112, USGPO, Washington, D.C. #1724—00395, 1975.

31. Rioch, M.J., Elke, S.C., Flint, A.A. et al., "NIMH Pilot Study in Training Mental Health Counselors," *Amer. J. of Orthopsychiat.* 33:678—689, 1963.

32. Sobey, F., *The Nonprofessional Revolution in Mental Health*, Columbia University Press, New York, 1970.

33. Bloom, B.L., "Human Accountability in a CMHC: Report on an Automated System," *Community Mental Health J.* 8:251—252, 1972.

34. Langsley, D.G. and Barter, J.T., "Treatment in the Community or State Hospital: An Evaluation," *Psychiatric Annals* 5:5, 62—70 (May) 1975.

35. Rodgers, C.W. and Doidge, J.R., "Is NIMH's Dream Coming True? Wyoming Centers Reduce State Hospital Admissions," *Community Mental Health J.* (in press).

36. Schmidt, L.J., "Reducing Reliance on the Psychiatric Hospital: The Utah Experience," *Psychiatric Annals* 5:5, 62—70 (May) 1975.

37. Dyck, D., "The Effect of a CMHC Upon State Hospital Utilization," *Am. J. of Psychiat.* 131:4, 453—456 (Apr.) 1974.

38. Lewin, K., "Group Decision and Social Change," in Newcomb, T.M. and Hartley, E.L. (eds.), *Readings in Social Psychology*, Henry Holt, New York, pp. 330—344, 1947.

39. Ozarin, L.D. and Spaner, F.E., "Mental Health Corporations, A New Trend in Providing Services," *Hosp. and Community Psychiatry*, 25:4, 225—227 (Apr.) 1974.

40. Schiff, S.K., "Community Accountability and Mental Health Services," *Mental Hygiene*, 54:2, p. 205—214 (Apr.) 1970.

41. Whitaker, L., "Social Reform and the CMHC: The Model Cities Experiment," *Amer. J. of Public Health* 60:10, 2003—2010 (Oct.) 1970.

42. Brown, B.S., Forword to *The Community Mental Health Center, Strategies and Programs*, edited by Beigel, A. & Levenson, A., Basic Books, New York, 1972.

43. Deutsch, A., *op. cit.*, p. 425.

44. Ochberg, F.M. and Brown, B.S., "Mental Health and the Law: Partners in Advancing Human Rights," *U. of Pa. Law Review* 123:2 491—508, (Philadelphia) (Dec.) 1974.

45. *Dixon v. Weinberger*, Civil Action #74—285, Robinson decision, Dec. 23, 1975.

46. Stone, A.A., "Overview: The Right to Treatment—Comments on the Law and Its Import," *Amer. J. of Psychiat.* 132:11, 1125—1134 (Nov.) 1975.

47. *Rouse v. Cameron*, 373 F 2d 451, D.C. Cir., 1966.

48. *Wyatt v. Stickney*, 325 F Supp. 481 (MD Ala. 1971).

49. *Wyatt v. Stickney*, 344 F Supp. 373, 376, 379, 385 (MD Ala. 1972).

50. *Burnham v. Dept. of Public Health*, 349 Supp. 1335 (ND Ga. 1972).

51. O'Connor v. Donaldson, 43 USLW, 4929 (1975).

52. Zusman, J., *Program Evaluation & Quality Control in Progress in Community Mental Health*, Vol. III, *op cit.*

53. Lombillo, J.R., Kiresuk, T., and Sherman, R.E., "Evaluating a CMH Program, Contract Fulfillment Analysis," *Hospital & Community Psychiat.* 24:11, 760–762 (Nov.) 1973.

54. Ochberg, F., "CMHC Legislation: Flight of the Phoenix," *Amer. J. of Psychiat.* 133:1, 56–61 (Jan.) 1976.

55. Aristotle, *Poetics*, Hill & Wang, New York, 1961.

56. Erikson, E.H., *Childhood & Society*, 2nd ed., W.W. Norton, New York, 1963.

CHAPTER 1—LEIGHTON

1. Dohrenwend, B.P. and Dohrenwend, B.S., *Social Status and Psychological Disorder: A Casual Inquiry*, New York, John Wiley, 1969.

2. Essen-Moller, E., "Individual Traits and Morbidity in a Swedish Rural Population," *Acta Psychiatrica et Neurologica Scanadinavica*, Supplementum 100, 1956.

3. Grob, G.N., *Mental Institutions in America*, Social Policy in 1875, New York: The Free Press, 1973.

4. Hagnell, O., *A Prospective Study of the Incidence of Mental Disorder*, Svenska Boforlaget Bonniers, 1966.

5. Kety, S.S., Rosenthal, D., Wender, P.H., and Schulsinger, F., "The Types and Prevalence of Mental Illness in the Biological and Adoptive Families of Adopted Schizophrenics," *J. Psychiat. Res.* 6 (Suppl. 1): 345–362, 1968.

6. Leighton, D.C., Harding, J.S., Macklin, D.B., Macmillan, A.M., and Leighton, A.H., *The Character of Danger*, Psychiatric Symptoms in Selected Communities, Vol. III, The Stirling County Study of Psychiatric Disorder and Sociocultural Environment, New York, Basic Books, 1963.

7. Leighton, A.H., Lambo, A.T., Hughes, C.C., Leighton, D.C., Murphy, J.M., and Macklin, D.B., *Psychiatric Disorder Among the Yoruba*, A Report from the Cornell–Aro Mental Health Research Project in the Western Region, Nigeria, Ithaca, N.Y., Cornell University Press, 1963.

8. Murphy, J.M., Leighton, A.H., "A Community Mental Health Centre: 1952–1968" (in preparation, 1977).

9. Murphy, J.M., "Mental Illness and Mortality in a Community Population, 1952–1968" (in preparation, 1977).

10. Spitzer, R.L., Fleiss, J. "A Re-analysis of the Reliability of Psychiatric Diagnosis," *British Journal Psychiat.* 125: 341–347, 1974.

11. Wing, J.K., Cooper, J.E., Sartorius, N., *The Measurement and Classification of Psychiatric Symptoms*, Cambridge, England, Cambridge University Press, 1974.

CHAPTER 2—DOHRENWEND

Beiser, M., "A Psychiatric Follow-up Study of "Normal" Adults," *American Journal of Psychiatry* 127: 1464–1472, 1971.

Bloom, B.L., "The Medical Model, Miasma Theory, and Community Mental Health," *Community Mental Health Journal* 1:333–338, 1965.

Brown, G.W., "Meaning, Measurement, and Stress of Life Events," in B.S. Dohrenwend and B.P. Dohrenwend (eds.), *Stressful Life Events: Their Nature and Effects*, New York, John Wiley, 1974, pp. 217–243.

Bunney, W.E., as quoted in a report on the National Conference on Depressive Disorders, in *The Nation's Health*, Washington, D.C., American Public Health Association, November 1975, p.5.

Caplan, G., *Principles of Preventive Psychiatry*, New York, Basic Books, 1964.

Caplan, G. & Grunebaum, H., "Perspectives on Primary Prevention," *Archives of General Psychiatry*, 17: 331–346, 1967.

Cooper, B. & Morgan, H.G., *Epidemiological Psychiatry*, Springfield, Ill.: Charles C. Thomas, 1973.

Cowen, E.L., "Social and Community Interventions," *Annual Review of Psychology* 24: 423–472, 1973.

Dohrenwend, B.P., "Social Status and Psychological Disorder: An Issue of Substance and an Issue of Method," *American Sociological Review*, 31: 14–34, 1966.

_____ . "Psychiatric Disorder in General Populations: Problem of the Untreated Case," *American Journal of Public Health*, 60: 1052–1064, 1970.

_____ . "Problems in Defining and Sampling the Relevant Population of Stressful Life Events," in B.P. Dohrenwend and B.S. Dohrenwend (eds.), *Stressful Life Events: Their Nature and Effects*, New York, John Wiley, 1974, pp. 275–310.

_____ . "Sociocultural and Social-Psychological Factors in the Genesis of Mental Disorders," *Journal of Health and Social Behavior*, 16: 365–392, 1975.

Dohrenwend, B.P. & Dohrenwend, B.S., *Social Status and Psychological Disorder*, New York, John Wiley, 1969.

_____ . "Social and Cultural Influences on Psychopathology," *Annual Review of Psychology* 25: 417–452, 1974. (a).

_____ . "Psychiatric Disorders in Urban Settings," in S. Arieti, and G. Caplan (eds.), *American Handbook of Psychiatry, Volume II.* New York, Basic Books, 1974, pp. 426–446. (b).

_____ . "Sex Differences and Psychiatric Disorders," *American Journal of Sociology* (In press for May 1976 issue).

_____ . "The Conceptualization and Measurement of Stressful Life Events: An Overview of the Issues." In J.S. Straus, H.M. Babigian and M. Roff (Eds.), *Proceedings of Conference on Methods of Longitudinal Research in Psychopathology.* New York: Plenum, in press.

_____ . (Eds.), *Stressful Life Events: Their Nature and Effects.* New York, Wiley, 1974. (a).

_____ . "Overview and Prospects for Research on Stressful Life Events," in B.S. Dohrenwend and B.P. Dohrenwend (Eds.), *Stressful Life Events: Their Nature and Effects*, New York, John Wiley, 1974, pp. 313–331. (b).

Duhl, L.J., "Discussion of Dunham's Community Psychiatry: The Newest Therapeutic Bandwagon." *International Journal of Psychiatry* 1: 569–571, 1965.

Dunham, H.W., "Community Psychiatry: The Newest Therapeutic Bandwagon," *International Journal of Psychiatry* 1: 553–566, 1965.

Durkheim, E., *Suicide* (trans. by J.A. Spaulding and G. Simpson), Glencoe, Ill., Free Press, 1951.

Eastwood, M.R., *The Relation Between Physical and Mental Illness*, Toronto, University of Toronto Press, 1975.

Faris, R.E.L. and Dunham, H.W., *Mental Disorders in Urban Areas: An Ecological Study of Schizophrenia and Other Psychoses*, Chicago, Chicago University Press, 1939.

Gersten, J.C., Langner, T.S., Eisenberg, J.G., and Orzek, L., "Child Behavior and Life Events: Undesirable Change or Change per se?" in B.S. Dohrenwend and B.P. Dohrenwend (eds.), *Stressful Life Events: Their Nature and Effects*, New York, John Wiley, 1974, pp. 159–170.

Glass, A.J., "Introduction," in P.G. Bourne (ed.), *The Psychology and Physiology of Stress*, New York, Academic Press, 1969, pp. xiii–xxx.

Glidewell, J.C., "A Social Psychology of Mental Health," in S.E. Golann, and C. Eisdorfer (eds.), *Handbook of Community Psychology*, New York, Appleton-Century-Crofts, 1972, pp. 211–246.

Gottesman, I.I. and Shields, J., *Schizophrenia and Genetics: A Twin Study Vantage Point*, New York, Academic Press, 1972.

Grinker, R.R., and Spiegel, J.P., *Men Under Stress*, New York, McGraw-Hill, 1963.

Gruenberg, E.M., "The Epidemiology of Schizophrenia," in S. Arieti and G. Caplan (eds.), *American Handbook of Psychiatry*, Vol. II, New York, Basic Books, 1974, pp. 448–463.

Hagnell, O., *A Prospective Study of the Incidence of Mental Disorder*, Stockholm, Svenska Bokförlaget Norstedts-Bonniers, 1966.

Heston, L.L., "Psychiatric Disorders in Foster Home Reared Children of Schizophrenic Mothers," *British Journal of Psychiatry* 112: 819–825, 1966.

Hinkle, L.E., and Wolff, H.G., "Health and The Social Environment," in A.H. Leighton, J.A. Clausen, and R.N. Wilson (eds.), *Explorations in Social Psychiatry*, New York, Basic Books, 1957, pp. 105–137.

Jarvis, E., *Insanity and Lunacy in Massachusetts: Report of the Commission on Lunacy, 1855*, Cambridge, Mass., Harvard University Press, 1971.

Kessler, M., and Albee, G.W., "Primary Prevention," *Annual Review of Psychology* 26:557–591, 1975.

Klerman, G.L. and Barrett, J.E., "The Affective Disorders: Clinical and Epidemiological Aspects," in S. Gershon and B. Shropsin (eds.), *Lithium: Its Role in Psychiatric Research and Treatment*, New York, Plenum, 1973, pp 201–236.

Kolb, L.C., *Modern Clinical Psychiatry*, Philadelphia, W.B. Saunders, 1973.

Kramer, M., Rosen, B.M., and Willis, E.M., "Definitions and Distributions of Mental Disorders in a Racist Society," in C.V. Willie, B.M. Kramer and B.S. Brown (eds.), *Racism and Mental Health*, Pittsburgh, University of Pittsburgh Press, 1973, pp. 353–459.

Langner, T.S., "Some Problems of Interpretation and Method," in T.S. Langner and S.T. Michael, *Life Stress and Mental Health*, New York, Free Press, 1963.

Leighton, A.H., *My Name Is Legion: Foundations for a Theory of Man in Relation to Culture*, New York, Basic Books, 1959.

———. "Poverty and Social Change," *Scientific American* 212: 21–27, 1965.

Leighton, D.C., Harding, J.S., Macklin, D.B., Macmillan, A.M., and Leighton, A.H., *The Character of Danger*, New York, Basic Books, 1963.

Lipowski, Z.J., "Psychiatry of Somatic Diseases: Epidemiology, Pathogenesis, Classification," *Comprehensive Psychiatry* 16: 105–124, 1975.

Mazer, M., "People in Predicament: A Study in Psychiatric and Psychosocial Epidemiology," *Social Psychiatry* 9: 85–90, 1974.

N.Y. Times, August 3, 1975, p. 49B.

Paster, S., "Psychotic Reactions Among Soldiers of World War II." *Journal of Nervous and Mental Disease* 108: 54–66, 1948.

Raines, G.N., "Forword," in American Psychiatric Association Committee on Nomenclature and Statistics, *Diagnostic and Statistical Manual: Mental Disorders.* Washington, D.C., American Psychiatric Association, 1952, pp. v–xi.

Research Task Force of the National Institute of Mental Health, *Research in the Service of Mental Health: Summary Report*, Washington, D.C., DHEW Publication No. (ADM) 75–236, 1975.

Robins, L.N., *Deviant Children Grown Up*, Baltimore, Williams and Wilkins, 1966.

Rosenthal, D. and Kety, S.S. (eds.), *Transmission of Schizophrenia*, London, Pergamon, 1968.

Shepherd, M., Cooper, B., Brown, A.C., and Kalton, G.W., *Psychiatric Illness in General Practice*, London, Oxford University Press, 1966.

Silverman, C., *The Epidemiology of Depression*, Baltimore, Johns Hopkins Press, 1968.

Smith, M.B. and Hobbs, N., *The Community and the Community Mental Health Center*, Washington, D.C., American Psychological Association, 1966.

Srole, L., "Measurement and Classification in Socio-Psychiatric Epidemiology," Midtown Manhattan Study (1954) and Midtown Manhattan Restudy (1974), *Journal of Health and Social Behavior* 16: 347–364, 1975.

Srole, L., Langner, T.S., Michael, S.T., Opler, M.K., and Rennie, T.A.C., *Mental Health in the Metropolis*, New York, McGraw-Hill, 1962.

Susser, M.W., *Community Psychiatry: Epidemiology and Social Themes*, New York, Random House, 1968.

Swank, R.L., "Combat Exhaustion," *Journal of Nervous and Mental Disease* 109: 475–508, 1949.

Thoday, J.M. and Gibson, J.B., "Environmental and Genetical Contributions to Class Difference: A Model Experiment," *Science* 167: 990–992, 1970.

Wagonfeld, M.O., "The Primary Prevention of Mental Illness: A Sociological Perspective," *Journal of Health and Social Behavior* 13: 195–203, 1972.

WNET Channel 13, *The Thin Edge: Depression*, March 31, 1975.

CHAPTER 2—LANGNER, GERSTEN & EISENBERG

Achenbach, T.M., *Developmental Psychopathology*, New York, Ronald Press, 1974.

Andry, R.G., *Delinquency and Parental Pathology*, London, Methuen, 1960.

Bacon, H.K., Child, I.L., and Barry, H.A., "A Cross-Cultural Study of Correlates of Crime," *Journal of Abnormal and Social Psychology*, 1963, 66, 291–300.

Bandura, A. and Walters, R., *Adolescent Aggression*, New York, Ronald Press, 1959.

Bandura, A. and Walters, R., *Social Learning and Personality Development*, New York, Holt, Rinehart, & Winston, 1963.

Baruch, D.W., and Wilcox, J.A., "A Study of Sex Differences in Pre-School Children's Adjustment Coexistent with Interparental Tensions," *Journal of Genetic Psychology*, 1944, 64, 281–303.

Baumrind, D., "Child Care Practices Anteceding Three Patterns of Pre-School Behavior," *Genetic Psychology Monographs*, 1967, 75, 43–88.

Bayley, N., "Behavioral Correlates of Mental Growth: Birth to 36 Years," *American Psychology* 1968, 23, 1–17.

Becker, E., *The Denial of Death*, New York, Free Press, 1973.

Becker, W.C., Peterson, D.R., Hellmer, L.A., Shoemaker, D.J., and Quay, H.C., "Factors in Parental Behavior and Personality as Related to Problem Behavior in Children," *Journal of Consulting Psychology*, 1959, 23, 107–118.

Becker, W.C., Peterson, D.R., Luria, Z., Shoemaker, D.J., and Hellmer, L.A., "Relations of Factors Derived from Parent-Interview Ratings to Behavior Problems of Five-Year-Olds," *Child Development*, 1962, 33, 509–535.

Bennett, I., *Delinquent and Neurotic Children: A Comparative Study*, New York, McGraw-Hill, 1962.

Berkowitz, L., *Aggression: A Social Psychological Analysis.* New York, McGraw-Hill, 1962.

Biller, H.B., "Father Absence and the Personality Development of the Male Child," *Developmental Psychology*, 1970, 2, 181–201.

Bower, E.M., Shellhamer, T.A., and Daily, J.M., "School Characteristics of Male Adolescents who Later Became Schizophrenic," *American Journal of Orthopsychiatry*, 1960, 30, 712–729.

Bowlby, J. and Ainsworth, M., *Maternal Care and Mental Health*, Geneva, Penguin, 1964.

Burnham, D., National Crime Panel Surveys, Law Enforcement Association, Administrative Justice Department, as cited in *New York Times*, April 15, 1974, pp. 1, 51.

Burt, C., *The Young Delinquent*, New York, Appleton, 1929.

Clausen, J.A. and Kohn, M.L., "Social Relations and Schizophrenia: A Research Report and a Perspective, in *The Etiology of Schizophrenia*, D.D. Jackson (ed.), New York, Basic Books, 1960.

Coleman, R.W. and Province, S., "Environmental Retardation (Hospitalism) in Infants Living in Families," *Pediatrics*, 1957, 19, 285–292.

Commoner, B., "A Reporter at Large (Energy-III)," *The New Yorker*, February 16, 1976, pp. 64–103.

Dohrenwend, B.P., "Sociocultural and Socio-Psychological Factors in the Genesis of Mental Disorders," *Journal of Health and Social Behavior*, 1975, 16, 365–392.

Dohrenwend, B.P., "Psychiatric Epidemiology as a Knowledge Base for Primary Prevention in Community Psychiatry and Community Mental Health." In *A Critical Appraisal of Community Psychiatry*, paper presented at the Symposium of the Kittay Scientific Foundation, New York, March 1976.

Douglas, J.W.B., *The Home and the School*, London, Macgibbon & Kee, 1964.

Douglas, J.W.B., "The School Progress of Nervous and Troublesome Children," *The British Journal of Psychiatry*, 1966, 112, 1115–1116.

Eisenberg, L., The Autistic Child in Adolescence, *American Journal of Psychiatry*, 1956, 112, 607–612.

Farina, A., Patterns of Role Dominance and Conflict in Parents of Schizophrenic Patients, *Journal of Abnormal and Social Psychology*, 1960, 61, 31–38.

Faris, R. and Dunham, H., *Mental Disorders in Urban Areas*. Chicago, Phoenix Press, 1965 (University of Chicago Press, 1939).

Fleiss, J.L., Spitzer, R.L., Endicott, J., and Cohen, J., "Quantification of Agreement in Multiple Psychiatric Diagnosis," *Archives of General Psychiatry*, 1972, 26, 168–171.

Garner, A.M. and Wenar, C., *The Mother-Child Interaction in Psychosomatic Disorders*. Urbana, University of Illinois Press, 1959.

Gersten, J.C., Langner, T.S., Eisenberg, J.G., and Simcha-Fagan, O., "Spontaneous Recovery and Incidence of Psychological Disorder in Urban Children and Adolescents," *Psychiatry Digests*, August 1975, 35–43.

Gersten, J.C., Langner, T.S., Eisenberg, J.G., Simcha-Fagan, O., & McCarthy, E.D., "Stability and Change in Children's and Adolescents' Disturbed Behaviors in a Longitudinal Study," *Journal of Abnormal Child Psychology*, 1976 (in press).

Glidewell, J.C., "Studies of Mothers' Reports of Behavior Symptoms in Their Children," in *The Definition and Measurement of Mental Health*, S.B. Sells (ed.), U.S. Public Health Statistics, Washington, D.C., Government Printing Office, 1968.

Glueck, S. and Glueck, E., *Unraveling Juvenile Delinquency*, New York, Commonwealth Fund, 1950.

Gooch, S. and Kellmer-Pringle, M.L., *Four Years on*. The National Bureau for Co-operation in Child Care, London, Longmans, Green, 1966.

Heston, L.L. "Psychiatric Disorders in Foster Home Reared Children of Schizophrenic Mothers," *British Journal of Psychiatry*, 1966, 112 (489), 819–825.

Hetherington, E.M. and Deur, J., "Effects of Father Absence on the Personality Development of Daughters," Unpublished manuscript, University of Wisconsin, 1970.

Hetherington, E.M., Stouwie, R.J., and Ridberg, E.H., "Patterns of Family Interaction and Child-Rearing Attitudes Related to Three Dimensions of Juvenile Delinquency," *Journal of Abnormal Psychology*, 1971, 78, 160–176.

Hughes, C.C., Tremblay, M., Rapoport, R.N., and Leighton, A.H., *People of Cove and Woodlot: Communities from the Viewpoint of Social Psychiatry*, Vol. II, The Stirling County Study of Psychiatric Disorder and Sociocultural Environment, New York, Basic Books, 1960.

Hunt, J. McV., *Intelligence and Experience*, New York, Ronald Press, 1961.

Jarvis, E., *Insanity and Lunacy in Massachusetts: Report of the Commission on Lunacy, 1855*, Cambridge, Harvard University Press, 1971.

Jenkins, R.L., "Psychiatric Syndromes in Children and Their Relation to Family Background," *American Journal of Orthopsychiatry*, 1966, 36, 450–457.

Jenkins, R.L. and Boyer, A., "Types of Delinquent Behavior and Background Factors," *International Journal of Social Psychiatry*, 1968, 14, 65–76.

Kanner, L., "Autistic Disturbance of Affective Contact," *Nervous Children*, 1943, 2, 217–250.

Kanner, L., "Follow-up Study of Eleven Autistic Children Originally Reported in 1943," *Journal of Autism and Childhood Schizophrenia*, 1971, 1, 119–145.

Kanner, L., Rodriquez, A., and Ashenden, B., "How Far Can Autistic Children Go in Matters of Social Adaptation?," *Journal of Autism and Childhood Schizophrenia*, 1972, 2, 9–33.

Kellam, S.G. and Schiff, S.K., "Adaptation and Mental Illness in the First-Grade Classroom of an Urban Community," Psychiatric Research Report 21, American Psychiatric Association, *Poverty and Mental Health*, January 1967, 79–91.

Kellmer-Pringle, M.L., Butler, N.R., and Davie, R., *11,000 Seven-Year-Olds*, The National Child Development Study, London, Longmans, Green, 1966.

Kessler, M. and Albee, G.W., "Primary Prevention," *Annual Review of Psychology*, 1975, 26, 557–591.

Langner, T.S., "A Twenty-Two Item Screening Score of Psychiatric Symptoms Indicating Impairment," *Journal of Health and Human Behavior*, 1962, 3, 269–276.

Langner, T.S., "Psychophysiological Symptoms and Women's Status in Two Mexican Communities," in *Approaches to Cross-Cultural Psychiatry*, J.M. Murphy and A.H. Leighton (eds.), Ithaca, N.Y., Cornell University Press, 1965, 360–392.

Langner, T.S., Gersten, J.C., and Eisenberg, J.G., "Approaches to Measurement and Definition in the Epidemiology of Behavior Disorders: Ethnic Background and Child Behavior," *International Journal of Health Services*, 1974, 4 (3), 483–501.

Lapouse, R. and Monk, M.A., "An Epidemiological Study of Behavior Characteristics in Children," *American Journal of Public Health*, 1958, 48, 1134–1144.

Lapouse, R. and Monk, M.A., "Behavior Deviations in a Representative Sample of Children: Variation by Sex, Age, Race, Social Class, and Family Size," *American Journal of Orthopsychiatry*, 1964, 34, 436–446.

Leighton, D.C., Harding, J.S., Macklin, D.B., Macmillan, A.M., and Leighton, A., *The Character of Danger*, the Stirling County Study of Psychiatric Disorder and Sociocultural Environment. III, New York, Basic Books, 1963.

Liverant, S., "MMPI Differences Between Parents of Disturbed and Non-Disturbed Children," *Journal of Consulting Psychology*, 1959, 23, 256–260.

Long, A., "Parents' Reports of Undesirable Behavior in Children," *Child Development*, 1941, 12, 43–62.

Lorr, M., "Classification of the Behavior Disorders," in *Annual Review of Psychology*. P.R. Farnsworth, O. McNemar, and Q. McNemar (eds.), Palo Alto, California, Annual Reviews, Inc., 1961.

MacFarlane, J.W., Allen, L., and Honzik, M.P., *A Developmental Study of the Behavior Problems of Normal Children Between Twenty-One Months and Fourteen Years*, Berkeley & Los Angeles, University of California Press, 1954.

McCord, W., McCord, J., and Zola, I.K., *Origins of crime*, New York, Columbia University Press, 1959.

McCord, W., McCord, J., and Howard, A., "Familial Correlates of Aggression in Non-Delinquent Male Children," *Journal of Abnormal and Social Psychology*, 1961, 62, 79−83.

McKeon, J., *Hierarchical Cluster Analysis*, Washington, D.C., George Washington University Biometrics Laboratory, 1967.

Mednick, S.A. and Schulsinger, F., "Studies of Children at High Risk for Schizophrenia," unpublished manuscript, New School for Social Research, 1972.

Merrill, M.A., *Problems of Child Delinquency*, Boston, Houghton Mifflin, 1947.

Mulligan, G., Douglas, J.W.B., Hammond, W.A., and Tizard, J., "Delinquency and Symptoms of Maladjustment: The Findings of a Longitudinal Study," *Proceedings of the Royal Society of Medicine*, 1963, 56, 1083−1086.

National Center for Health Statistics: Data from the National Health Survey, *Parent Ratings of Behavioral Patterns of Children, United States*, Vital and Health Statistics, U.S. Department of Health, Education, and Welfare Publications, 1971, No. (HSM) 72−1010, Series 11 (108).

National Institute of Mental Health, *Outpatient Psychiatric Clinics Annual Statistical Report*, Washington, D.C.: Public Health Service Publication 1854, 1966.

Read, K.H., "Parents' Expressed Attitudes and Children's Behavior," *Journal of Consulting Psychology*, 1945, 9, 95−100.

Robins, L.N., *Deviant Children Grown Up*. Baltimore, Williams & Wilkins, 1966.

Robins, L.N., and Lewis, R.G., "The Role of the Antisocial Family in School Completion and Delinquency: A Three-Generation Study," *Sociological Quarterly*, 1966, 7, 500−514.

Rosenthal, M.J., Finkelstein, M., Ni, E., and Robertson, R.E., "A Study of Mother-Child Relationships in the Emotional Disorders of Children," *Genetic Psychology Monographs*, 1959, 60, 65−116.

Rosenthal, M.J., Ni, E., Finkelstein, M., and Berkwits, G.K., "Father-Child Relationships and Children's Problems," *AMA Archives of General Psychiatry*, 1962, 7 (5), ____

Rosenthal, D., "A Program of Research on Heredity in Schizophrenia," in S.A. Mednick, F. Schulsinger, J. Hipping, and B. Bell *Genetics, Environment and Psychopathology*, 1974.19

Rutter, M., Tizard, J., and Whitmore, K. (eds.), *Education, Health, and Behavior*. London, Longman, 1970.

Sears, R.R., Whiting, J.W.M., Nowlis, V., and Sears, P.S., "Some Child-Rearing Antecedents of Aggression and Dependency in Young Children," *Genetic Psychology Monographs*, 1953, 47, 135−234.

Sears, R.R., Maccoby, E.E., and Levin, H., *Patterns of Child-Rearing*, New York, Harper, 1957.

Sears, R.R., "Relation of Early Socialization Experiences to Aggression in Middle Childhood," *Journal of Abnormal and Social Psychology*, 1961, 63, 466−492.

Shaw, C.R. and McKay, H.D., *Juvenile Delinquency and Urban Areas*, Chicago, University of Chicago Press, 1942.

Shaefer, E.S., "A Circumplex Model for Maternal Behavior," *Journal of Abnormal and Social Psychology*, 59, 1959, 226—235.

Shields, J. and Slater, E., "Heredity and Psychological Abnormality," in *Handbook of Abnormal Psychology*, H.J. Eysenck (ed.), New York, Basic Books, 1961.

Shepherd, M., Oppenheim, B., and Mitchell, S., *Childhood Behavior and Mental Health*, New York, Grunet Stratton, 1971.

Skeels, H.M., "Headstart on Headstart: 30-year evaluation," Fifth Annual Distinguished Lecturer in Special Education, Summer Session 1966, Los Angeles, U.S.C. School of Education, 1967.

Spitz, R., "Anaclitic Depression: An Inquiry into the Genesis of Psychiatric Conditions in Early Childhood," *Psychoanal. Study of the Child* 1946, 2, 313—342.

Stein, Z. and Susser, M., "Mutability of Intelligence and Epidemiology of Mild Mental Retardation," *Review of Educational Research*, 1970, 40 (1), 29—66.

Stein, Z.A. and Susser, M.W., "Changes Over Time in the Incidence and Prevalence of Mental Retardation, *Exceptional Infant*, Vol. 2, Studies in Abnormalities, J. Hellmuth (ed.), New York, Brunner/Mazel, 1971.

Stouffer, S.A. (ed.), *The American Soldier*, Princeton, Princeton University Press, 1950.

Thomas, A., Chess, S., and Birch, H., "The Origins of Personality," *Scientific American*, 1970, 223, 102—109.

Tuddenham, R.D., Brooks, J., and Milkovich, L., "Mothers' Reports of Behavior of Ten-Year-Olds: Relationships with Sex, Ethnicity, and Mother's Education," *Developmental Psychology*, 1974, 10 (6), 959—995.

White, S.H., Day, M.L., Freeman, P.K., Hartman, S.A., and Messenger, K.P., *Federal Programs for Young Children: Review and Recommendations. I*, Washington, D.C., Government Printing Office, 1973.

Yolles, S.F. and Kramer, M., "Vital Statistics," in *The Schizophrenic Syndrome*, L. Bellak & L. Loeb (eds.), New York, Grune & Stratton, 1969, pp. 66—113.

Zubin, J., Salzinger, K., Fleiss, J.L., Gurland, B., Spitzer, R.L., Endicott, J., and Sutton, S., "Biometric Approach to Psychopathology: Abnormal and Clinical Psychology. Statistical, Epidemiological, and Diagnostic Approaches," *Annual Review of Psychology*, 1975, 26, 621—671.

CHAPTER 2—STRUENING

Brandon, R.N., "Differential Use of Mental Health Services: Social Pathology or Class Victimization?" in Guttentag, M., and Struening, E.L. (eds.), *Handbook of Evaluation Research*, Vol. II., Beverly Hills, Calif., Sage Publications, 1975.

Cassel, J., "Social Science in Epidemiology, Psychosocial Processes and Stress Theoretical Formulation," in Struening, E.L. and Guttentag, M. (eds.), *Handbook of Evaluation Research*, Vol. 1. Beverly Hills, Calif., Sage Publications, 1975.

Cassel, J.C. and Leighton, A.H., "Epidemiology and Mental Health," in Goldston, S.E. (ed.), *Mental Health Considerations in Public Health*. U.S. Department of Health, Education, and Welfare, Public Health Service, Health Services and Mental Health Administration, National Institute of Mental Health, Washington, D.C., October 1969.

Cobb, S., "A Model for Life Events and Their Consequences," in Dohrenwend, B.S. and Dohrenwend, B.P. (eds.), *Stressful Life Events: Their Nature and Effects*, New York: John Wiley, 1974.

Gersten, J.C., Langner, T.S., Eisenberg, J.G., Simcha-Fagan, O., and McCarthy, E.D., "Stability and Change in Types of Behavioral Disturbance of Children and Adolescents," *Journal of Abnormal Child Psychology 4* (2): 111–127, 1976.

Mechanic, D., "Discussion of Research Programs on Relations Between Stressful Life Events and Episodes of Physical Illness," in Dohrenwend, B.S. and Dohrenwend, B.P. (eds.), *Stressful Life Events: Their Nature and Effects*, New York: John Wiley, 1974.

Rabkin, J.G. and Struening, E.L., "Social Change Stress and Illness: A Selective Literature Review," *Psychoanalysis and Contemporary Science* (in press).

Ryan, W. (ed.), *Distress in the City*, Cleveland, Press of Case Western Reserve, 1969.

Selye, H., *The Stress of Life*, rev. ed., New York: McGraw-Hill, 1976.

Spitzer, R. and Wilson, P.T., "Nosology and the Official Psychiatric Nomenclature," in Friedman, A., Kaplan, H. and Sadock, B. (eds.), *Comprehensive Textbook in Psychiatry*, Vol. I., Baltimore, Williams and Wilkins, 1975.

Struening, E.L., "Social Area Analysis as a Method of Evaluation," in Struening, E.L. and Guttentag, M. (eds.), *Handbook of Evaluation Research*, Vol. I., Beverly Hills, Calif., Sage Publications, 1975.

Thomas, C.S. and Garrison, V., "A General Systems View of Community Mental Health," in Bellak, L. and Barten, H. (eds.), *Progress in Community Mental Health*, Vol. III, New York, Brunner/Mazel, 1975.

CHAPTER 3—MOSHER

1. Joint Commission on Mental Illness and Health, *Action for Mental Health: Final Report of the Joint Commission on Mental Illness and Health 1961*, New York, Basic Books, 1961.

2. Chu, F.D. and Trotter, S., *The Madness Establishment*, New York, Grossman, 1974.

3. Glick, I., Hargreaves, W.A., and Goldfield, M.D., "Short vs. Long Hospitalization: A Prospective Controlled Study, I: The preliminary results of a one-year follow-up of schizophrenics," *Archives of General Psychiatry*, 30:363–369, 1974.

4. Wilson, H., "Conventional Psychiatric Treatment: A Dispatching Process," unpublished draft report, 1975.

5. Gunderson, J.G. and Mosher, L.R., "The Cost of Schizophrenia," *American Journal of Psychiatry* 132(9):901–906, 1975.

6. Fairweather, W., Sanders, D., Cressler, D., and Maynard, H., *Community Life for the Mentally Ill: An Alternative to Institutional Care*, Chicago, Aldine Publishing, 1969.

7. Pasamanick, D., Scarpitti, F., and Dimitz, S., *Schizophrenics in the Community: An Experimental Study in the Prevention of Hospitalization*, New York, Appleton-Century-Crofts, 1967.

8. Langsley, O., Pittman, F. III, and Swank, G., "Family Crisis in Schizophrenics and Other Mental Patients," *Journal of Nervous and Mental Diseases* 149:270–276, 1969.

9. Fairweather, G.W., Sanders, D.H., Tornatzky, L.G., with Harris, R.N., *Creating Change in Mental Health Organizations*, New York, Pergamon Press, 1974.

10. Taube, C.A. and Redick, R.W., "Recent Trends in the Utilization of Mental Health Facilities," in Zusman, J. and Bertsch, E.F. (eds.), *The Future Role of the State Hospital*, Lexington, Mass., Lexington Books, 1975.

11. Almond, R., *The Healing Community: Dynamics of the Therapeutic Milieu*, New York, Jason Aronson, 1974.

12. Brill, H. and Malzberg, B., Statistical report based on the arrest record of 5354 male ex-patients released from New York state mental hospitals during the period 1946–8, unpublished report, 1954.

CHAPTER 3–TISCHLER

1. NIMH, *Community Mental Health Center Program Operating Handbook*, Part I: Policy and Standards Manual, U.S. Department of Health, Education and Welfare, September 1, 1971.

2. Mechanic, D., *Mental Health and Social Policy*, Englewood Cliffs, New Jersey, Prentice Hall, 1969.

3. Myers, J.K., Lindenthal, J., Pepper, M., "Life Events and Psychiatric Impairment," *J. Nerv. Ment. Dis.* 152:149–157, 1971.

4. Macmillan, A.M., "The Health Opinion Survey: Technique for Estimating Prevalence of Psychoneurotic and Related Types of Disorder in Communities," *Psychological Reports* 3: 325–339, 1957.

5. Guerin, G., Venoff, J., and Feld, S., Americans View Their Mental Health. New York, Basic Books, 1960.

6. Andersen, R., Kravits, J., and Anderson, O.W., *Equity in Health Services*, Cambridge, Mass., Ballinger, 1975.

7. Tischler, G.L., "Development of Standards for Evaluating Direct Patient Care," in Riedel, D.C., Tischler, G.L., Myers, J.K., (eds.), *Patient Care Evaluation in Mental Health Programs.* Cambridge, Mass., Ballinger, 1974.

8. Goldblatt, P., Brauer, L., Garrison, V., Henisz, J., and Malcolm-Lawes, M., "A Chart Review Checklist for Utilization Review in a Community Mental Health Center," *Hosp. Comm. Psychiatry* 24: 753–756, 1973.

9. Raskin, A., Schulterbrandt, J., and Reatig, N., "Factors of Psychopathology in Interview, Ward Behavior and Self-report Ratings of Hospitalized Depressives," *J. Consult. Psychol.* 31: 270–278, 1967.

10. Katz, M.M., Lyerly, S.B., "Methods for Measuring Adjustment and Social Behavior in the Community," *Psychological Reports* 13: 503–535, 1963.

11. Tischler, G.L., Henisz, J.E., Myers, J.K., and Garrison, V., "Catchmenting and the Use of Mental Health Services," *Arch. Gen. Psychiatry* 27: 389–392, 1972.

12. Tischler, G.L., Henisz, J.E., Myers, J., and Garrison, V., "The Impact of Catchmenting," *Administration in Mental Health* 1: 22–29, 1972.

13. Henisz, J.E., Tischler, G.L., and Myers, J.K., "Epidemiologic and Ecologic Analyses," in Riedel, D.C., Tischler, G.L. and Myers, J.K., (eds.), *Patient Care Evaluation in Mental Health Programs*, Cambridge, Mass., Ballinger, 1974.

14. Tischler, G.L., Henisz, J.E., Myers, J.K., and Boswell, P.C., "Utilization of Mental Health Services: I. Patienthood and the Prevalence of Symptomatology in the Community," *Arch. Gen. Psychiatry* 32: 412–416, 1975.

15. Tischler, G.L., Henisz, J.E., Myers, J.K., and Boswell, P.C., "Utilization of Mental Health Services: II. Mediators of Service Allocation," *Arch. Gen. Psychiatry* 32: 416–418, 1975.

16. Tischler, G.L., Aries, E., Cytrynbaum, S., and Wellington, S.W., "The Catchment Area Concept," in Bellak, L. and Barten, H.H. (eds.), *Progress in Community Mental Health*, Vol. III, New York, Brunner/Mazel, 1975.

CHAPTER 3—ELLSWORTH

1. Arnhoff, F.N., "Social Consequences of Policy Toward Mental Illness," *Science* 18: 1277–1281, 1975.

2. Cronbach, L.J. and Furdy, L., "How We Should Measure Change—Or Should We?" *Psychological Bulletin* 74: 68–90, 1970.

3. DuBois, P.H., *Multivariate Correlation Analysis*, New York, Harper, 1957.

4. Ellsworth, R.B., *PARS V Community Adjustment Scale*, Institute for Program Evaluation, Box 4654, Roanoke, Va. 24015, 1974.

5. Ellsworth, R.B., "Consumer Feedback in Measuring the Effectiveness of Mental Health Programs," in M. Guttentag & E.L. Struening (eds.), *Handbook of Evaluation Research*, Beverly Hills, Calif., Sage Publications, 1975.

6. Erickson, R.C., "Outcome Studies in Mental Hospitals, a Review," *Psychological Bulletin* 82: 519–540, 1975.

7. Evenson, R.C., "Community Adjustment Changes Following Psychiatric Inpatient Care," presented at the 83rd annual meeting of the American Psychological Association, Chicago, August 1975.

8. Fontana, A.F. and Dowds, B.M., "Assessing Treatment Outcome: I Adjustment in the Community," *Journal of Nervous and Mental Diseases* 161: 221–230, 1975.

9. Hogarty, G.E., "Drug and Sociotherapy in the Aftercare of Schizophrenic Patients," *Arch. of Gen. Psychiatry* 81: 609–618, 1974.

10. Hollingshead, A.B. and Redlich, F.C., *Social Class and Mental Illness*, New York, John Wiley, 1958.

11. Lord, F.M., "Elementary Models for Measuring Change," in C.W. Harris (ed.), *Problems in Measuring Change*, Madison, University of Wisconsin Press, 1962.

12. Luborsky, L., "Clinician's Judgments of Mental Health," *Arch. Gen. Psychiatry* 7: 407–417, 1962.

13. May, P.R.A., *Treatment of Schizophrenia*, New York, Science, 1969.

14. Pasamanick, B., Scarpitti, F.R., and Dinitz, S., *Schizophrenics in the Community*, New York, Appleton-Century-Crofts, 1967.

15. Riessman, F., Cohen, J., and Pearl, A., *Mental Health and the Poor*, New York, The Free Press of Glencoe, 1964.

16. Rosenhan, D.L., "On Being Sane in Insane Places," *Science* 179: 250–258, 1973.

17. Waskow, I.E. and Parloff, M.B., "Psychotherapy Change Measures," DHEW Publication #(ADM) 74–120, Superintendent of Documents, Washington, D.C. 20402, 1975.

18. Zlotowski, M. and Cohen, D., "Effects of Change in Hospital Organizations Upon the Behavior of Psychiatric Patients," presented at meeting of Eastern Psychological Association, Atlantic City, April 1965.

CHAPTER 3—KIRESUK AND LUND

Chu, F.D. and Trotter, S., *The Madness Establishment: Ralph Nader's Study Group Report on the National Institute of Mental Health*, New York, Grossman, 1974.

Davis, H.R., "Change and Innovation," in *Administration in the Mental Health Services*, Saul Feldman (ed.), Springfield, Ill., Charles C. Thomas, 1973.

Davis, H.R. and Salasin, S., "Improving the Policy Relevance of Social Research and Development," prepared for the National Academy of Sciences Study Project on Social Research and Development, Laurence Lynn (ed.), 1975.

Garwick, G., "Guide To Goals I," unpublished technical aid, Minneapolis, Program Evaluation Project, 1973.

Glaser, E.M., "Knowledge Transfer and Institutional Change," *Professional Psychology* 4: 434–444, 1973.

Jones, S. and Garwick, G., "Guide To Goals Study: Goal Attainment Scaling as Therapy Adjunct?" *P.E.P. Newsletter*, July–August, 4(6), 1–3.

Kiresuk, T.J. and Sherman, R.E., "Goal Attainment Scaling: A General Method For Evaluating Comprehensive Community Mental Health Programs," *Community Mental Health Journal* 4: 443–453, 1968.

LaFerriere, L. and Calsyn, R., "Goal Attainment Scaling: An Effective Treatment Technique in Short Term Therapy," unpublished report, Michigan State University, 1975.

Lynn, L. and Salasin, S., "Human Services: Should We, Can We Make Them Available to Everyone?" *Evaluation*, Spring 1974, 4–6.

Scriven, M., "The Methodology of Evaluation," in *Perspectives of Curriculum*, Ralph W. Tyler, Robert M. Gagne, and Michael Scriven (eds.), AERA Monograph Series on Curriculum Evaluation, no. 1. Chicago, Rand McNally, 1967.

Sherman, R.E., "Content Validity Argument for Goal Attainment Scaling," unpublished report, Minneapolis, Program Evaluation Resource Center, 1975.

Sherman, R.E., Baxter, J., and Audette, D., "An Examination of the Reliability of the Kiresuk-Sherman Goal Attainment Score by Means of Components of Variance," unpublished report, Minneapolis, Program Evaluation Resource Center, 1974.

Smith, D.L., "Goal Attainment Scaling as an Adjunct to Counseling," *Journal of Counseling Psychology* 23(1): 22–27, 1976.

Rogers, E.M., *Diffusion of Innovations*, New York, Free Press, 1962.

Zaltman, G., Duncan, R., and Holbek,J., *Innovations and Organization*, New York, John Wiley, 1973.

CHAPTER 3-GLICK

1. Glick, I.D., Hargreaves, W.A., and Goldfield, M.D., "Short vs. Long Hospitalization: A Prospective Controlled Study, I, The Preliminary Results of a One-Year Follow-up of Schizophrenics," *Arch. Gen. Psychiatry* 30: 363–369, 1974.

2. Glick, I.D., Hargreaves, W.A., Raskin, M. et al., "Short versus Long Hospitalization: A Prospective Controlled Study, II, Results for Schizophrenic Inpatients," *Am. J. Psychiatry* 132: 385–390, 1975.

3. Glick, I.D., Hargreaves, W.A., Drues, J. et al., "Short vs. Long Hospitalization: A Prospective Controlled Study, III, Inpatient Results for Nonschizophrenics," *Arch. Gen. Psychiatry* 33: 78–83, 1976.

4. Glick, I.D., Hargreaves, W.A., Drues, J., and Showstack, J.A., "Short versus Long Hospitalization: A Prospective Controlled Study, IV, One-year Follow-up Results for Schizophrenic Patients," *Am. J. Psychiatry* 133: 509–514, 1976.

5. Glick, I.D., Hargreaves, W.A., Drues, J., and Showstack, J.A., "Short versus Long Hospitalization: A Prospective Controlled Study, V, One-year Follow-up Results for Nonschizophrenic Patients," *Am. J. Psychiatry* 133: 515–517, 1976.

CHAPTER 4-KLERMAN

1. Arnhoff, F.N., "Social Consequences of Policy Toward Mental Illness," *Science*, 1277–1281, 1975.

2. Brown, G.W., Bone, M., Dalison, B., and Wing, J.K., *Schizophrenia and Social Care*, London, Oxford University Press, 1966.

3. Caffey, J.R., Jones, R.D., Burton, E., Diamond, L.S., and Bowen, W.T., "A Controlled Study of Brief Hospitalization for Schizophrenics," Veterans Administration, Cooperative Studies in Psychiatry, Central Neuropsychiatric Research Laboratory, Perry Point, Maryland, 1967.

4. Cole, J.O., Goldberg, S., and Klerman, G.L., "Phenothiazine Treatment in Acute Schizophrenia," *Arch. Gen. Psych.* 10: 246–261, 1964.

5. Crane, G.E., "Two Decades of Psychopharmacology and Community Mental Health: Old and New Problems of the Schizophrenic Patient," *Transactions of the N.Y. Acad. Sciences* 36: 644–656, 1974.

6. Davis, J.M., "Overview: Maintenance Therapy in Psychiatry: I. Schizophrenia," *Am. J. Psych.* 12: 1237–1295, 1975.

7. Fairweather, G.E., Sanders, D.H., Cressler, D.L., and Maynard, H., "Community Life for the Mentally Ill," Chicago, Aldine, 1969.

8. Garmezy, N., "Children at Risk: The Search for the Antecedents of Schizophrenia, Part II: Ongoing Research Programs, Issues, and Intervention," *Schizophrenia Bulletin*, 9: 55–125, 1974.

9. Glick, I.D., Hargreaves, W.A., Drues, J., and Schostack, J.A., "Short versus Long Hospitalization: A Prospective Controlled Study, IV, One Year Follow-up Results for Schizophrenic Patients," *Am. J. Psych.* 133:509–514, 1976.

10. Goffman, E., *Asylums*, New York, Doubleday, 1961.

11. Goldstein, M.J., "Premorbid Adjustment, Paranoid Status, and Patterns of Response to Phenothiazine in Acute Schizophrenia," *Schizophrenia Bulletin* 3:24–37, 1970.

12. Greenblatt, M., Solomon, M., Evans, A.S., and Brooks, G.W., (eds.), "Drugs and Social Therapy in Chronic Schizophrenia," Springfield, Ill., Charles Thomas, 1965.

13. Greenblatt, M., "Historical Forces Affecting the Closing of Mental Hospitals" in: *NIMH Proceedings of Conference on Closing of State Mental Hospitals.* Menlo Park, Stanford Research Institute, 1974.

14. Gruenberg, E.M. (ed.), "Evaluating the Effectiveness of Community Mental Health Services," *Milbank Memorial Fund Q.* Part 2, Vol. 44, January 1966.

15. Herz, M.I., Endicott, J., Spitzer, R.L., and Mesnikoff, A., "Day Versus Inpatient Hospitalization: A Controlled Study," *Am. J. Psych.* 127:1371–1382, 1971.

16. Herz, M.I., Endicott, J., and Spitzer, R.L., "Brief Hospitalization of Patients With Families: Initial Results," *Am. J. Psych.* 132:413–418, 1975.

17. Hogarty, G.E., "The Plight of Schizophrenics in Modern Treatment Programs," *Hosp. and Comm. Psych.* 22:197–203, 1971.

18. Hogarty, G.E., Goldberg, S.C., "Drugs and Sociotherapy in the After-care of Schizophrenic Patients: One-Year Relapse Rates," *Arch. Gen. Psych.* 28:54–64, 1973.

19. Khan, N., "Follow-up of Patients After Closing of Grafton State Hospital," unpublished manuscript, Commonwealth of Massachusetts Department of Mental Health, 1975.

20. Klerman, G.L., "Current Evaluation Research on Mental Health Services," *Am. J. Psych.* 131:783–787, 1974.

21. _____ . "Behavior Control and the Limits of Reform," *Hastings Center Report* 5:40–45, 1975.

22. _____ . "Better But Not Well: Social and Ethical Issues in the Deinstitutionization of the Mentally Ill," presented at the Conference on Alternatives to Incarceration, sponsored by the Behavior Control Research Group, Hastings Center, Hastings-on-Hudson, N.Y., May 1976.

23. Klerman, G.L. and Barrett, J.E., unpublished data, 1976.

24. Kraft, A., Binner, P., Truitt, E., and Morton, W.D., "The Psychiatric Care Systems' Silent Minority," *Am. J. Psych.* 128:26–30, 1976.

25. Kramer, M., "Applications of Mental Health Statistics: Uses in Mental Health Programs of Statistics Derived From Psychiatric Services and Selected Vital and Morbidity Records," Geneva, World Health Organization, 1969.

26. Kramer, M., "Population Change of Schizophrenia, 1970–1985," presented at Second Rochester International Conference on Schizophrenia," Rochester, N.Y., May 1976.

27. Laing, R.D., in Romano, J. (ed.), *The Origins of Schizophrenia*, Amsterdam, Excerpta Medica Foundation, 1967.

28. Langfeldt, G., "The Schizophrenic States," Copenhagen, E. Munksgaard, 1939.

29. Leff, J.P. and Wing, J.K., "Trial of Maintenance Therapy in Schizophrenics," *Brit. Med. J.* 2: 599–604, 1971.

30. Mosher, L.R., Matthews, S., and Menn, A., "Soteria: A New Treatment for Schizophrenia—One Year Follow-up Data," *Am. J. Orthopsych.* 44: 207–208, 1974.

31. Pasamanick, B., Scarpitti, F.R., and Dinitz, S., *Schizophrenics in the Community: An Experimental Study in the Prevention of Hospitalization*, New York, Appleton-Century-Crofts, 1967.

32. Reidel, D.C., Brauer, L., Brenner, M.H., Goldblatt, P., Schwartz, C., Myers, J.K., and Klerman, G.L., "Developing a System for Utilization Review and Evaluation in Community Mental Health Centers," *Hosp. & Comm. Psych.* 32:1221, 1975.

33. Rodnick, E.H., "Antecedents and Continuities in Schizophreniform Behavior," in Dean, S.R. (ed.) *Schizophrenia: The First Ten Dean Award Lectures*, New York, MSS Information Corp., 1973.

34. Rosenhan, D.L., "On Being in Insane Places," *Science* 179: 250–258, 1973.

35. Schwartz, C., Myers, J.K., and Astrachan, B.M., "Concordance of Multiple Assessments of the Outcome of Schizophrenia," *Arch. Gen. Psych.* 32: 1221, 1975.

36. Siegler, M. and Osmond, H., "Models of Madness, Models of Medicine," New York, McMillan, 1974.

37. Smith, W.G., Kaplan, J., and Siker, D., "Community Mental Health and the Seriously Disturbed Patient," *Arch. Gen. Psych.* 30: 693–696, 1974.

38. Spitzer, R.L., "On Pseudoscience in Science, Logic in Remission, and Psychiatric Diagnosis: A Critique of Rosenhan's 'On Being Sane in Insane Places,'" *J. Abnorm. Psychol.* 84: 442–452, 1975.

39. Venables, P.H., "Partial Failure of Cortical-Subcortical Integration as a Factor Under-lying Schizophrenic Behavior" in Romano, J. (ed.), *The Origins of Schizophrenia*, Amsterdam, Excerpta Medica Foundation, 1967.

40. Weisman, G., Feirstein, A., and Thomas, C., "Three-day Hospitalization— A Model for Intensive Intervention," *Arch. Gen. Psych.* 21: 620–629, 1969.

41. Zwerling, I. and Wilder, J.F., "Day Hospital Treatment of Psychotic Patients," *Curr. Psychiat. Ther.* 2: 200–210, 1962.

CHAPTER 4—SERBAN

Angst, J., Zur Atiologie und Nosologie endogener depressiver Psychosen, Springer-Verlag, Berlin-Heidelberg, 1966.

Astrup, C., Fossum, A., and Holmboe, R., *Prognosis in Functional Psychosis*, Springfield, Ill., Charles C. Thomas, 1962.

Birley, J.L.T. and Brown, G.W., "Crises and Life Changes Preceding the Onset or Relapse of Acute Schizophrenia: Clinical Aspects," *British Journal of Psychiatry* 116: 327–333, 1970.

Dohrenwend, B.S., "Life Events as Stressors: A Methodological Inquiry," *Journal of Health and Social Behavior* 14: 167–175, 1974.

Epstein, S. and Coleman, M., "Drive Theories of Schizophrenia," *Psychosomatic Medicine* 32: 114–141, 1970.

Gittelman-Klein, R. and Klein, D., "Premorbid Asocial Adjustment and Prognosis in Schizophrenia," *Journal of Psychiatric Research* 7: 35–53, 1969.

Higgins, J., "Process-reactive Schizophrenia," *Journal of Nervous and Mental Disease* 149: 451–471, 1969.

Hollingshead, A.B. and Redlich, F.C., *Social Class and Mental Illness: A Community Study*, New York, John Wiley, 1958.

Holmes, T.H. and Rahe, R.H., "The Social Readjustment Rating Scale," *Journal of Psychosomatic Research* 11: 213–217, 1967.

Langfeldt, G., "The Prognosis in Schizophrenia," *Acta Psychiatrica et Neurological Scandinavica, Supplementation*, 110, Copenhagen, 1956.

Lagner, T.S. and Michel, S.T., *Life Stress and Mental Health*, The Midtown-Manhattan Study, New York, The Free Press, 1963.

Magaro, P.A., "A Validity and Reliability Study of the Process-reactive Self-report Scale," *Journal of Consulting and Clinical Psychology* 32: 482–485, 1969.

Michaux, W.W., Katz, M., Kurland, A.A., and Gansereit, K.H., *The First Year Out*, Baltimore, Johns Hopkins Press, 1969.

Phillips, L., "Case History Data and Prognosis in Schizophrenia," *Journal of Nervous and Mental Disease* 117: 515–523, 1953.

Serban, G., "Stress in Schizophrenics and Normals," *British Journal of Psychiatry* (May) 126, 1975.

Serban, G., "Functioning Ability in Schizophrenics and Normals: Short-term Prediction for Rehospitalization of Schizophrenics," *Compre. Psychiatry* 16: 5, 1975.

Serban, G. and Gidynski, C., "Differentiating Criteria for Acute-Chronic Distinction in Schizophrenia," *Arch. Gen. Psychiatry* 32: 705–712, 1975.

Serban, G., Gidynski, C., and Zimmerman, A., "The Role of Informants in Community Oriented Mental Health Programs for Schizophrenics," *Diseases of the Nervous System* 4: 36, 1975.

Serban, G. and Thomas, A., "Attitudes and Behaviors of Acute and Chronic Schizophrenic Patients Regarding Ambulatory Treatment," *Amer. J. Psychiatry* 131: 9, 1974.

Serban, G., "Parental Stress in the Development of Schizophrenic Offspring," *Comm. Psychiatry* 16, 1975.

Serban, G. and Gidynski, C., "Schizophrenic Patients in Community," *New York State Journal of Medicine* 74: 11, 1974.

Stephens, J.H. and Astrup, C., "Prognosis in 'Process' and 'Non-process' Schizophrenia," *American Journal of Psychiatry* 126: 498–503, 1969.

Taube, A.C. and Readlich, R., "Utilization of Mental Health Resources by Persons Diagnosed with Schizophrenia," *NIMH Statistical Report*, May 1972.

Turner, R.J. and Zabo, L.J., "Social Competence and Schizophrenic Outcome: An Investigation and Critique," *Journal of Health and Social Behavior* 9: 41–51, 1968.

Ullmann, L.P. and Giovannoni, J.M., "The Development of a Self-report Measure of the Process-reactive Continuum," *Journal of Nervous and Mental Disease* 138: 38–41, 1964.

Vaillant, G.E., "Prospective Prediction of Schizophrenic Remission," *Arch. Gen. Psychiatry* 11:509–517, 1964.

Wallis, G.G., "Stress as a Predictor in Schizophrenia," *British Journal of Psychiatry* 120: 375–384, 1972.

Watson, C.G. and Logue, P.E., "A Note on the Interjudge Reliability of Phillips and Elgin Scale Ratings," *Journal of Clinical Psychology* 24: 66–68, 1968.

Wittman, P. and Steinberg, L., "Follow-up of an Objective Evaluation of Prognosis in Dementia Praecox and Manic-Depressive Psychosis," *Elgin State Hospital Papers* 5: 216–227, 1964.

Zigler, E. and Phillips, L., "Social Competence and Outcome in Psychiatric Disorder," *Journal of Abnormal and Social Psychology* 63: 264–271, 1961.

CHAPTER 4–CARPENTER

1. Davis, J.M., "Overview: Maintenance Therapy in Psychiatry: I, Schizophrenia," *Amer. J. Psychiatry* 132: 1237–1245, 1975.

2. Doherty, J.P., "Maintenance Phenothiazine Treatment in Schizophrenia: A Review," presented to American Psychiatric Association, Miami, 1976.

3. Strauss, J.S. and Carpenter, W.T., "The Prediction of Outcome in Schizophrenia, I: Characteristics of Outcome," *Arch. Gen. Psychiatry* 27: 739–746, 1972.

4. Strauss, J.S. and Carpenter, W.T., Prediction of Outcome in Schizophrenia III: Five-Year Outcome and Its Predictors, "A Report from the International Pilot Study of Schizophrenia," *Arch. Gen. Psychiatry* (in press), 34:159–163, 1977.

5. Schwartz, C.C., Myers, J.K., and Astrachan, B.M., "Concordance of Multiple Assessments of the Outcome of Schizophrenia: On Defining the Dependent Variable in Outcome Studies," *Arch. Gen. Psychiatry* (in press).

6. Engelhardt, D.M., *Psychiatric News*, 1974, cited in "Pharmacotherapy with Schizophrenics," *Physician*, pp. 27–31, September 4, 1974.

7. Carpenter, W.T., McGlashan, T.H., and Strauss, J.S., "The Treatment of Acute Schizophrenia Without Drugs: An Investigation of Some Current Assumptions," *Am. J. Psychiat.* (in press), 134:14–20, 1977.

8. Gardos, G. and Cole, J., "Maintenance Antipsychotic Therapy: Is the Cure Worse Than the Disease?" *Amer. J. Psychiatry* 133: 32–36, 1976.

9. Goldstein, M.J., "Premorbid Adjustment, Paranoid Status, and Patterns of Response to Phenothiazine in Acute Schizophrenia," *Schizophrenia Bulletin* 3: 24–37, 1970.

10. Leff, J.P. and Wing, J.K., "Trial of Maintenance Therapy in Schizophrenics," *Brit. Med. J.* 2:599–604, 1971.

11. Klein, D.F., "Who Should Not Be Treated with Neuroleptics, But Often Are," in *Rational Psychopharmacotherapy and The Right to Treatment* (Ch. 3), Frank J. Ayd, Jr. (ed.), Ayd Medication Communications, Baltimore, 1974, pp. 29–36.

12. Lamb, H. and Goertzel, V., "Discharged Mental Patients—Are They Really in the Community?" *Arch. Gen. Psychiatry* 24:29–34, 1971.

13. Kohn, M., "The Interaction of Social Class and Other Factors in the Etiology of Schizophrenia," *Am. J. Psychiatry* 133(2): 177–180, 1976.

14. Strauss, J.S. and Carpenter, W.T., Jr., "The Prediction of Outcome in Schizophrenia, II, Relationships Between Predictor and Outcome Variables: A Report From The WHO International Pilot Study of Schizophrenia," *Arch. Gen. Psychiatry* 31: 37–42, 1974.

CHAPTER 4—GRUENBERG

1. American Public Health Association, Program Area Committee on Mental Health, *Mental Health Disorders: A Guide to Control Methods*, New York, APHA, 1962.

2. Barton, R., *Institutional Neurosis*, Bristol, England, John Wright and Sons, 1966.

3. Congress of the United States, Mental Retardation Facilities and Community Mental Health Centers Act of 1963, Public Law 88–164, *U.S. Federal Register* 54.201205, 1964, pp. 5951–5956.

4. Gruenberg, E.M., "Benefits of Short-Term Hospitalization," in Cancro, R., Fox, N., and Shapiro, L.E., *Strategic Intervention in Schizophrenia: Current Developments in Treatment*, New York, Behavioral Publications, 1974.

5. _____. "Obstacles to Optimal Psychiatric Service Delivery Systems," *Psychiatric Quarterly* 46:483–496, 1972.

6. Gruenberg, E.M. and Huxley, J., "Mental Health Services Can Be Organized to Prevent Chronic Disability," *Community Mental Health Journal* 6:431–436, 1970.

7. Gruenberg, E.M., Snow, H.B., and Bennett, C.L., "Preventing the Social Breakdown Syndrome," in Redlich, F.C., *Social Psychiatry*, Baltimore, Williams & Wilkins, 1969.

8. Hunt, R.C., Gruenberg, E.M., Hacken, E., and Huxley, M., "A Comprehensive Hospital-Community Service in a State Hospital," *Amer. J. Psychiatry* 117(9):817–821, March 1961.

9. Kasius, R.V., "The Social Breakdown Syndrome in a Cohort of Long-Stay Patients in the Dutchess County Unit, 1960–63," in Gruenberg, E.M. (ed.), *Evaluating the Effectiveness of Community Mental Health Services*, New York, Mental Health Materials Center, 1966.

10. Macmillan, D., "Hospital-Community Relationships," in *An Approach to the Prevention of Disability from Chronic Psychoses*, New York, Milbank Memorial Fund, 1958.

11. New York State Department of Mental Hygiene, Community Mental Health Services Act, Chapter 10 of the Laws of 1954, as amended by Chapters 145 and 805 of the Laws of 1954. (Article 8–A in Mental Hygiene Law and General Orders, Utica, New York).

12. Turns, D. and Gruenberg, E.M., "Social Breakdown Syndrome vs. Institutional Neurosis." Paper presented at the New Research Program, American Psychiatric Association, Annual Meeting, Honolulu, May 9, 1973.

Index

About the Editor

George Serban, M.D., Principal Researcher at the New York University Medical Center, has dedicated a part of his time to clinical research on schizophrenia focusing on the adjustment of the schizophrenics in the community. At this time he continues his studies of stress experienced by schizophrenics living in the community. He has published the results of his research in various scientific journals.